# Cancer-Us:
## *A Comprehensive Journey Through the History, Treatment, and Global Impact of Cancer*

By Rabbi Michael Schoening

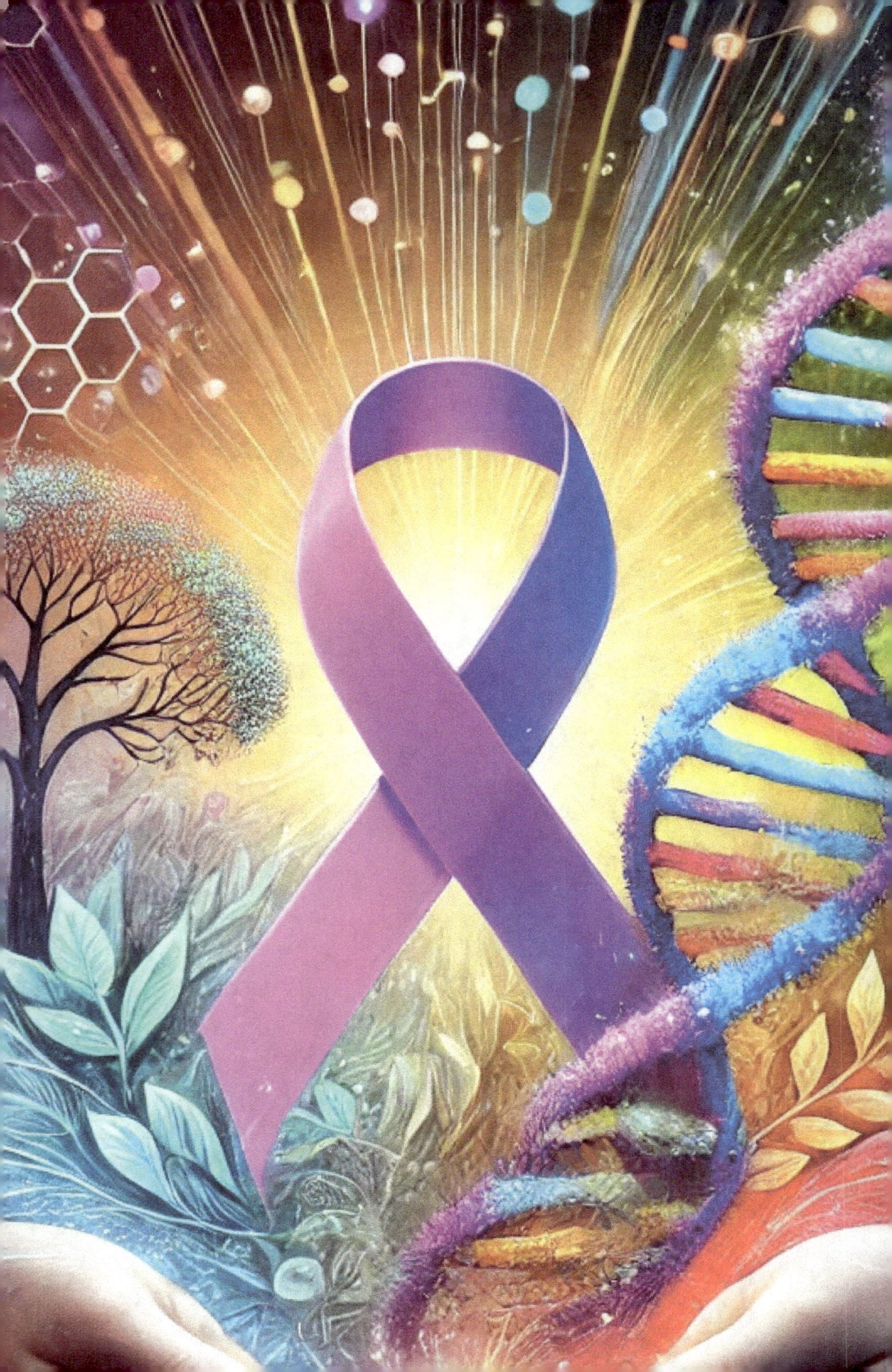

A compilation text by Rabbi Michael Schoening. Dedicated to my younger brother Chris who survived cancer, to all who didn't, to their families, and to humanity; may we cure ourselves from within.

*Cancer-Us* is an in-depth exploration of one of humanity's most formidable adversaries: cancer. From its earliest historical records to cutting-edge treatments of today, this book takes readers on a journey through the science, stories, and societal impact of this disease.

The book reveals the complexities of cancer, examining its origins, causes, and treatments, while delving into the global disparities in healthcare access. It features an exhaustive directory of every known type of cancer, from the common to the rare, detailing their causes, treatments, and global prevalence. Alongside the science, it highlights personal stories of survival, resilience, and innovation, weaving together a narrative of hope and determination.

Blending Western medical advancements with traditional and natural approaches, *Cancer-Us* challenges readers to think critically about prevention, treatment, and the medical industry's role. This book is a resource, a call to action, and a beacon of hope for patients, caregivers, and advocates worldwide.

Table of Contents

Part I: Introduction
1. Foreword
2. Cancer and Society: The Great Equalizer
3. Why Write This Book? Personal Connections and the Larger Picture
4. Disclaimers and Scope: A Rabbi's Perspective on Cancer

Part II: The History of Cancer
1. Ancient Beginnings: The First Accounts of Cancer
2. The Evolution of Cancer Theories: From Humors to Modern Science
3. Milestones in Cancer Treatment: Surgery, Radiation, and Beyond
4. The Role of Advocacy and Awareness in Modern Times

Part III: The Cancer Industry
1. Profits vs. Patients: Unpacking the Controversy
2. Big Pharma and the Quest for a Cure
3. Insurance, Access, and the Cost of Care Worldwide
4. Conspiracy Theories: Does the Industry Want Us Sick?

5.　The Role of Advocacy Organizations and Charities

Part IV: The Cancers A-Z Directory
　　1.　An Exhaustive Directory: Every Known Cancer
　　2.　Alphabetical Entries (A-Z): Causes, Treatments, and Global Perspectives

Part V: Global Theories, Treatments, and Cures
　　1.　Western Medicine's Approach: The Science of Cancer
　　2.　Eastern Medicine: Balancing Energy and Healing Holistically
　　3.　Indigenous and Natural Cures: Insights from Around the World
　　4.　The Rise of Immunotherapy and Precision Medicine
　　5.　Global Disparities in Treatment and Prevention

Part VI: Prevention and Advocacy
　　1.　The Role of Lifestyle: Diet, Exercise, and Stress Management
　　2.　Vaccination and Screening Programs: Game Changers in Prevention
　　3.　How Governments, NGOs, and Communities Can Make a Difference

    4.   Empowering Patients and Caregivers: Knowledge as Power

Part VII: Personal Stories of Hope
    1.   Survivors: Stories of Courage and Determination
    2.   Caregivers: The Unsung Heroes
    3.   Innovators and Researchers: The Minds Behind the Breakthroughs

Part VIII: Conclusion
    1.   Lessons Learned: The State of Cancer Research and Advocacy Today
    2.   The Path Forward: A Vision for a Cancer-Free Future

Part IX: References and Resources
    1.   Academic Studies and Scientific Literature
    2.   Global Health Organizations and Databases
    3.   Support Groups and Advocacy Networks
    4.   Further Reading: Books, Documentaries, and Articles

Introduction: The Cancer Conundrum

Cancer is one of humanity's oldest adversaries, a shadow that looms large in every corner of the world. It touches lives indiscriminately—young and old, rich and poor, those who live in bustling cities and those in remote villages. Despite centuries of study and countless advances in medicine, cancer remains a formidable challenge.

This book is born out of a personal connection to cancer and a deep commitment to understanding it. My brother was diagnosed with non-Hodgkin's lymphoma—a moment that forever changed my perception of life and mortality. His journey, filled with both uncertainty and resilience, sparked a relentless curiosity in me. As a Rabbi, I have dedicated my life to studying the complexities of human experience, searching for meaning, and offering guidance in times of crisis. Cancer, I realized, is not just a medical issue; it is a spiritual, emotional, and societal one.

Yet, as I delved deeper into the world of cancer, I was struck by unsettling questions: Why do cancer rates continue to rise despite decades of research? Why are some treatments unaffordable or inaccessible? Is there a cure for cancer that has yet to reach the people who need it most—or worse, one that is deliberately suppressed?

These questions led me on a journey through the labyrinth of cancer—its history, biology, treatments, and the industries that have grown around it. *Cancer-Us* is the result of this journey: a book that seeks to educate, empower, and provoke thought.

In these pages, you will find:
- A comprehensive exploration of the many types of cancer, including their causes, treatments, and prevention.
- Global perspectives on how cancer is treated, viewed, and understood across cultures.
- Stories of resilience and hope from patients, caregivers, and medical professionals.
- Investigations into the economic and ethical questions surrounding cancer care.
- Practical insights into prevention and navigating life with cancer.

This book does not claim to have all the answers. I am not a doctor, nor do I claim medical expertise. What I bring is a deep respect for knowledge, a hunger for truth, and a desire to make complex topics accessible to everyone. I hope this book becomes a companion for anyone touched by cancer—a guide to understanding, a source of hope, and perhaps, a spark for change.

Preface: Why Write This Book?

Cancer is more than a disease; it is a mirror reflecting the state of our health, our systems, and our society. It is a personal struggle and a global challenge.

For centuries, cancer has been viewed as an enemy to be defeated. From ancient Egypt to modern laboratories, humans have waged war against this disease. Yet, cancer is also a teacher, revealing the limits of our understanding and the resilience of the human spirit.

My brother's battle with Non-Hodgkin's lymphoma brought cancer into sharp focus for me. I watched him endure treatments that were as taxing as the disease itself, but I also witnessed his incredible strength and the power of hope. His recovery was a victory, but it left me with lingering questions: Why does cancer still claim so many lives? Why are some treatments available to a select few? How can we, as a society, do better?

As I researched and reflected, I realized that cancer is not just a medical issue; it is intertwined with economics, culture, environment, and ethics. For every breakthrough in treatment, there are stories of inequity and hardship. For every promising therapy, there are patients who cannot afford it.

This book is my attempt to bring together the threads of knowledge, stories, and perspectives on cancer. It is a tribute to those who fight, a resource for those who seek understanding, and a challenge to the systems that profit from suffering.

Chapter 1: What Is Cancer?

Cancer is not a single disease but a collection of diseases that share a common trait: the uncontrolled growth of abnormal cells. While this may sound simple, cancer is one of the most complex and challenging conditions to understand and treat. It touches every aspect of human life — physical, emotional, and societal.

But cancer is more than just a medical condition. It is a story about the fragility of life, the resilience of the human body, and the limits of our knowledge. To truly understand cancer, we must explore its biology, causes, and the profound impact it has on individuals and communities around the world.

The Biology of Cancer: Cells Gone Rogue

Every human body is made up of trillions of cells, each performing specific tasks that sustain life. These cells operate under a set of rules encoded in their DNA. Cells grow, divide, and die in a controlled manner, a process critical to maintaining the balance of the body. When this system works correctly, it allows the body to heal injuries, replace old cells, and adapt to changing environments.

Cancer begins when these rules are broken. A single cell experiences a mutation — an error in its DNA — that disrupts its normal function. Instead of dying when it's supposed to, this cell begins to grow and divide uncontrollably. Over time, these abnormal cells form a mass called a tumor, which can invade nearby tissues and, in some cases, spread to distant parts of the body through the bloodstream or lymphatic system. This process is known as metastasis and is what makes cancer so dangerous.

Tumors can be classified as:
- Benign: Non-cancerous tumors that do not invade other tissues.
- Malignant: Cancerous tumors that grow aggressively and spread to other parts of the body.

Cancer's ability to adapt and evade the body's defenses makes it particularly challenging to treat. For example, some cancer cells can hide from the immune system, while others develop resistance to chemotherapy or radiation.

Why Does Cancer Happen?

The causes of cancer are as diverse as the disease itself. Scientists have identified several factors that contribute to the development of cancer, including genetic mutations, environmental exposures, and lifestyle choices.

Genetic Mutations

Mutations in DNA are at the heart of cancer. Some mutations are inherited from parents, which is why people with a family history of certain cancers, like breast or colon cancer, have a higher risk. For example:
- BRCA1 and BRCA2: Mutations in these genes significantly increase the risk of breast and ovarian cancer.
- Lynch Syndrome: A genetic condition associated with an increased risk of colorectal and endometrial cancers.

Other mutations occur spontaneously during a person's life. These can be caused by external factors, such as exposure to carcinogens, or simply by the natural wear and tear of DNA over time.

Environmental Factors

The environment plays a significant role in cancer risk. Certain substances, known as carcinogens, can damage DNA and lead to cancer. Examples include:
- Tobacco Smoke: Responsible for 85-90% of lung cancer cases.
- Radiation: Ultraviolet (UV) rays from the sun cause skin cancers like melanoma.

- Industrial Chemicals: Workers exposed to asbestos are at high risk for mesothelioma, a rare cancer of the lung lining.

In addition, environmental factors like air and water pollution have been linked to higher cancer rates in some communities.

Viruses and Infections

Some cancers are caused by viruses or other infectious agents that alter DNA. Notable examples include:
- Human Papillomavirus (HPV): Linked to cervical, throat, and anal cancers.
- Hepatitis B and C Viruses: Major contributors to liver cancer.
- Epstein-Barr Virus (EBV): Associated with certain lymphomas and nasopharyngeal cancer.

Vaccination programs, like the HPV vaccine, have been instrumental in reducing cancer risk in populations around the world.

Lifestyle Choices

Certain habits and behaviors can significantly impact cancer risk. For example:
- Diet: Diets high in processed foods, red meat, and sugar are linked to colon and stomach cancers. Conversely, diets rich in fruits, vegetables, and whole grains are protective.
- Physical Activity: Regular exercise lowers the risk of several cancers, including breast and colon cancer.
- Alcohol and Tobacco: Excessive alcohol consumption and smoking are leading causes of cancer worldwide.

Studies show that up to 40% of cancer cases could be prevented through lifestyle changes, making prevention a critical area of focus.

The Global Impact of Cancer

Cancer is not just a disease of the individual—it is a global crisis. In 2020 alone, there were an estimated 19.3 million new cancer cases and nearly 10 million deaths worldwide. Cancer does not discriminate, but its prevalence and impact vary significantly by region.

Cancer Hotspots Around the World
- Australia: The highest rates of skin cancer due to high UV exposure and a

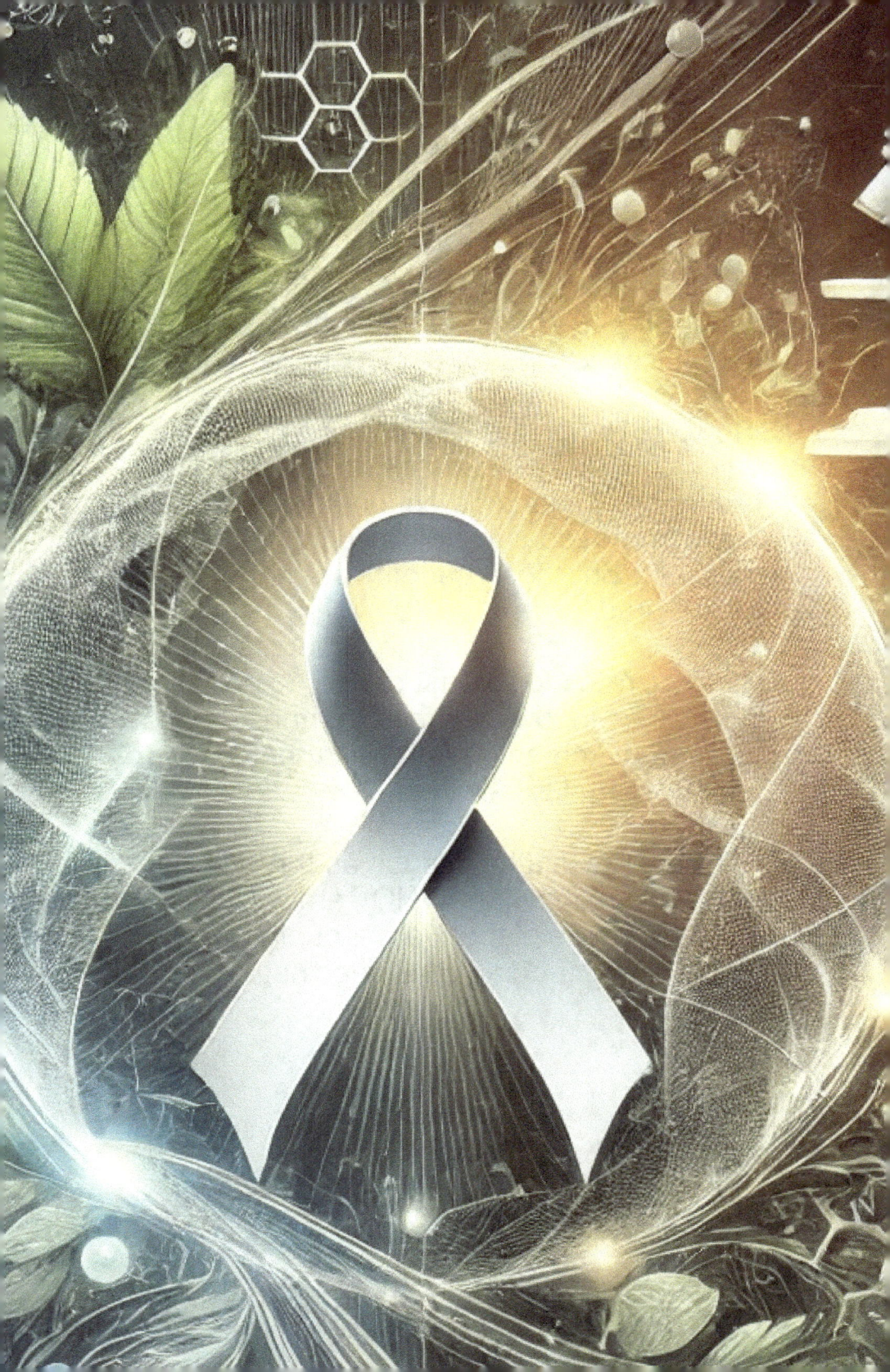

predominantly fair-skinned population.
- Southeast Asia: Liver cancer is prevalent due to widespread Hepatitis B and C infections.
- Western Countries: High rates of lung, breast, and colorectal cancers due to diet, lifestyle, and longer lifespans.

Survival Rates and Disparities

Advances in early detection and treatment have improved survival rates for many cancers, but these benefits are not equally distributed.
- In high-income countries, 5-year survival rates for breast cancer exceed 90%.
- In low-income countries, lack of access to screening and treatment leads to higher mortality.

Global organizations, such as the World Health Organization (WHO), are working to address these disparities through awareness campaigns, funding, and vaccination programs.

A Human Perspective on Cancer

Cancer affects more than the body—it profoundly impacts every aspect of a person's life. For patients, the diagnosis is often accompanied by fear, uncertainty, and a sense of isolation. For families, it is a time of emotional upheaval, as they juggle caregiving responsibilities with their own grief and hope.

One patient described her battle with cancer as "a war I didn't sign up for, but one I had to fight." For another, cancer was a "wake-up call" that inspired him to live more fully, despite the challenges of treatment.

These stories remind us that cancer is not just a biological disease; it is a deeply human experience.

Why Understanding Cancer Matters

By understanding cancer, we gain the tools to fight it. Knowledge empowers us to make informed decisions about prevention, seek early detection, and advocate for equitable access to care. This book is an effort to demystify cancer and explore its complexities, offering hope and practical insights to everyone affected by it.

Chapter 2: The History of Cancer

Cancer is not a modern disease. It has existed as long as humanity itself, documented in ancient texts and seen in the remains of our ancestors. From its mysterious beginnings to the groundbreaking discoveries of today, the history of cancer is a story of human curiosity, resilience, and ingenuity. Understanding where we've been in the fight against cancer offers critical insights into where we are headed.

Ancient Beginnings: The Earliest Evidence of Cancer

The first evidence of cancer comes from ancient remains, with fossilized bones showing signs of tumors. Researchers have found signs of cancer in Egyptian mummies dating back to 3000 BCE, confirming that even in the absence of modern pollutants, cancer existed. However, without advanced tools for diagnosis, ancient societies could only observe and speculate about the disease.

The Ebers Papyrus: The First Medical Record

One of the earliest written references to cancer is found in the Ebers Papyrus, an ancient Egyptian medical text from around 1500 BCE. The document describes tumors of the breast and suggests cauterization as a treatment. The absence of further suggested remedies implies that ancient Egyptians viewed cancer as incurable.

Cancer in Ancient Greece: The Origin of the Name

The term "cancer" has its roots in ancient Greece. The physician Hippocrates (460-370 BCE), often called the "Father of Medicine," described tumors as "karkinos," the Greek word for crab. He likely chose this name because the spread of cancerous growths resembled the legs of a crab. Hippocrates believed cancer resulted from an imbalance in the body's four humors: blood, phlegm, yellow bile, and black bile. This theory persisted for over a millennium, shaping how cancer was understood and treated.

Medieval Misconceptions and Stagnation

The Middle Ages saw little progress in cancer understanding. Religious interpretations often dominated medical thought, with cancer viewed as a punishment for sins or a test of faith. Treatments included prayers, herbal remedies, and bloodletting, none of which addressed the disease effectively.

## Avicenna and Medical Advancements in the Islamic Golden Age

During the Islamic Golden Age (8th to 14th centuries), the Persian physician Avicenna made significant contributions to medicine through his comprehensive text, *The Canon of Medicine.* Avicenna described surgical techniques for removing tumors and emphasized early detection. Though these ideas were advanced for their time, the understanding of cancer's causes and mechanisms remained limited.

## The Renaissance: A Shift Toward Observation

The Renaissance ushered in an era of scientific curiosity and observation, laying the groundwork for modern medicine. Anatomical studies by figures like Andreas Vesalius (1514–1564) revealed detailed structures of the human body, challenging long-held beliefs. However, cancer was still poorly understood, often attributed to an excess of "black bile," as per Hippocratic teachings.

## Surgical Advances

In the 16th and 17th centuries, surgery became a more common treatment for cancer. Surgeons like Ambroise Paré refined techniques for tumor removal, though without anesthesia or sterilization, these procedures were painful and often deadly. Despite their limitations, these efforts marked the beginning of a more systematic approach to treating cancer.

The Enlightenment: Cancer Meets the Microscope

The invention of the microscope in the 17th century revolutionized cancer research. Scientists like Antonie van Leeuwenhoek used this new tool to study tissues at the cellular level, providing the first glimpse into the microscopic world of cancer.

The Birth of Pathology

In 1775, British surgeon Percivall Pott linked scrotal cancer to chimney sweeps' exposure to soot, making it the first cancer identified with a specific environmental cause. This discovery was a landmark in understanding cancer as more than just a random affliction—it was the result of external factors.

## The 19th Century: Foundations of Modern Oncology

The 19th century brought significant advances in cancer diagnosis and treatment. Rudolf Virchow, a German physician and pathologist, is credited with founding modern pathology. His work demonstrated that cancer arises from changes in normal cells, laying the groundwork for the cellular theory of cancer.

## Surgical Triumphs and Limitations

Advances in anesthesia and sterilization made cancer surgeries more effective. The introduction of radical mastectomies by William Halsted in the late 1800s offered hope for breast cancer patients, though the procedures were invasive and disfiguring.

## The 20th Century: A Century of Breakthroughs

The 20th century transformed cancer research and treatment, driven by scientific discoveries and technological innovations

## The Discovery of Radiation Therapy

In 1895, Wilhelm Roentgen discovered X-rays, and within a decade, Marie Curie identified radium's ability to destroy cancerous tissue. These discoveries led to the development of radiation therapy, which became a cornerstone of cancer treatment.

## Chemotherapy: From War to Medicine

In the 1940s, scientists discovered that nitrogen mustard, a chemical weapon used in World War II, could kill rapidly dividing cells. This finding led to the development of the first chemotherapy drugs, which targeted cancer cells but also caused significant side effects.

## The Role of Viruses in Cancer

The link between viruses and cancer was established in the mid-20th century. Peyton Rous discovered the Rous sarcoma virus in chickens, earning a Nobel Prize and opening the door to understanding virus-induced cancers like those caused by HPV and Hepatitis B.

## The Genetic Revolution

The discovery of DNA's double helix by James Watson and Francis Crick in 1953 marked a turning point in cancer research. In the decades that followed, scientists identified specific genes, like oncogenes and tumor suppressor genes, that play key roles in cancer development.

## Targeted Therapies

The 21st century has seen the rise of targeted therapies, which attack cancer cells based on their unique genetic profiles. Drugs like imatinib (Gleevec), which treats chronic myeloid leukemia, represent a new era of precision medicine.

## The Present and Future: Toward a Cure

Today, cancer research is more advanced than ever. Breakthroughs in immunotherapy, which harnesses the immune system to fight cancer, offer new hope. CAR-T cell therapy, for example, has shown remarkable success in treating blood cancers.

## Global Collaboration

The fight against cancer is now a global effort. Organizations like the World Health Organization and the American Cancer Society fund research, promote awareness, and advocate for early detection and prevention.

Challenges Ahead

Despite progress, challenges remain. Cancer is not one disease but many, each with unique characteristics. The high cost of treatment and disparities in access to care continue to be major obstacles.

Conclusion: Lessons from History

The history of cancer is a testament to human ingenuity and perseverance. From ancient observations to cutting-edge therapies, each era has brought us closer to understanding and controlling this complex disease. By learning from the past, we can continue to innovate and bring hope to those affected by cancer.

Chapter 3: Cancer and Western Society

Cancer is not only a biological disease but also a societal one, deeply influenced by the environment, culture, economy, and lifestyle of the regions it touches. In Western societies, cancer has become a leading cause of death, reflecting the complex interplay between modern living and health. This chapter explores how lifestyle, industrialization, diet, stress, and environmental factors contribute to the prevalence of cancer in the West, while contrasting these trends with those in non-Western societies.

The Rise of Cancer in Western Society

A Disease of Modern Living?

Cancer has long been considered a disease of civilization. Ancient societies certainly experienced cancer, but its prevalence appears to have skyrocketed with industrialization and the modernization of daily life. This has led some researchers to label cancer a "disease of affluence," one tied closely to the advances and challenges of contemporary living.

In Western societies, cancer rates are higher than in many developing regions. Factors contributing to this rise include:

- Longevity: As people live longer, the likelihood of developing cancer increases. Many cancers are age-related, with the majority of cases occurring in individuals over 60.
- Lifestyle Factors: Sedentary lifestyles, diets high in processed foods, and widespread tobacco and alcohol use significantly increase cancer risk.
- Environmental Exposures: Industrial pollutants, pesticides, and urban air quality all contribute to the carcinogenic burden in Western countries.

Diet and Cancer: A Western Paradox

The Western Diet and Its Risks

The typical Western diet—characterized by high consumption of red meat, processed foods, sugar, and saturated fats—has been strongly linked to several types of cancer, including colorectal, breast, and stomach cancers. Processed meats, in particular, have been classified as Group 1 carcinogens by the World Health Organization (WHO), placing them in the same category as tobacco.

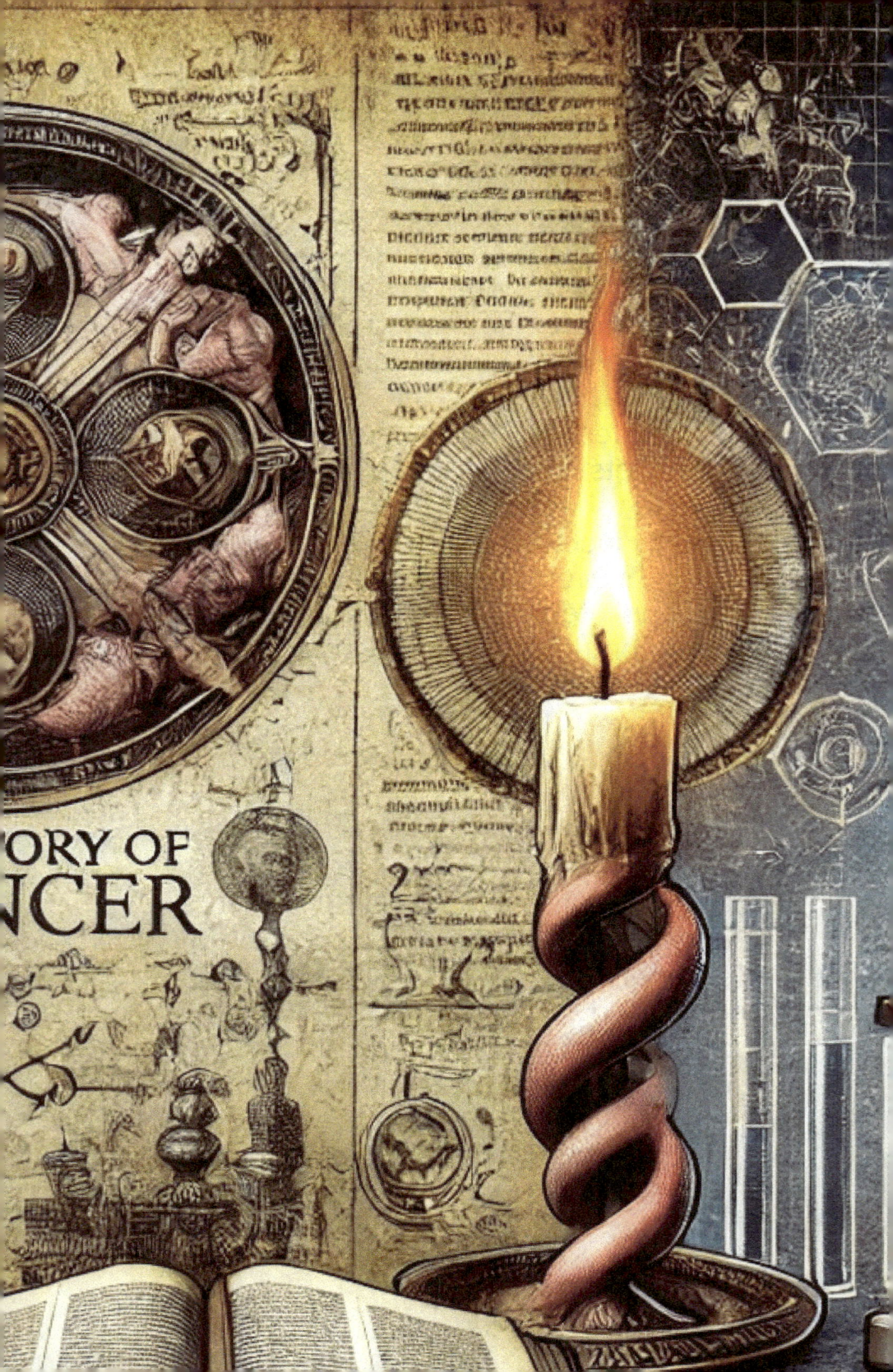

Studies also show that the Western diet is deficient in protective foods like fruits, vegetables, and whole grains. These foods are rich in antioxidants and fiber, which play a crucial role in reducing cancer risk by neutralizing free radicals and promoting healthy digestion.

The Obesity-Cancer Link

Obesity, a growing epidemic in Western nations, is a major risk factor for at least 13 types of cancer, including liver, kidney, pancreatic, and uterine cancers. Excess body fat promotes chronic inflammation and hormonal imbalances, creating an environment where cancer can thrive.

Contrast with Traditional Diets

In contrast, traditional diets like the Mediterranean diet or plant-based diets in non-Western societies are associated with lower cancer rates. For example:
• The Mediterranean diet, rich in olive oil, fish, and fresh produce, is linked to lower rates of breast and colorectal cancers.
• Japanese diets, which emphasize fish, rice, and fermented foods, are

associated with lower incidences of stomach cancer, despite high rates of salt consumption.

Environmental Carcinogens in the West

Industrialization and Pollution

The industrial revolution brought economic prosperity but also introduced new environmental hazards. Exposure to industrial chemicals, heavy metals, and pollutants has been linked to higher cancer rates.

Key examples include:
- Air Pollution: Studies show that long-term exposure to fine particulate matter increases the risk of lung cancer.
- Water Contamination: Carcinogens like arsenic and nitrates in water supplies have been linked to bladder and stomach cancers.
- Pesticides: Agricultural workers and communities near farmlands face higher rates of cancers like non-Hodgkin lymphoma due to pesticide exposure.

Urban vs. Rural Cancer Rates

Urban areas in Western societies tend to have higher cancer rates than rural areas. Contributing factors include:
- Higher levels of air and light pollution.
- Greater exposure to processed foods and sedentary lifestyles.
- Limited access to green spaces and physical activity opportunities.

Stress and Cancer: A Modern Epidemic

The Biology of Stress and Cancer

Chronic stress, common in fast-paced Western societies, may indirectly contribute to cancer development and progression. Stress hormones like cortisol can weaken the immune system, reduce the body's ability to repair DNA damage, and promote inflammation, creating a fertile ground for cancer.

Case Studies: Stress and Survival

Studies show that cancer patients with high stress levels often have worse outcomes than those who adopt stress-reducing practices like meditation, yoga, or counseling. Programs focusing on emotional well-being have been shown to improve survival rates and quality of life for cancer patients.

## Healthcare Systems and Cancer Outcomes

### Access to Screening and Early Detection

Western healthcare systems often emphasize early detection, which has improved survival rates for many cancers. Mammograms, colonoscopies, and other screening programs have significantly reduced deaths from breast, colorectal, and cervical cancers.

However, access to these resources is not universal. In the U.S., for example, individuals without insurance or living in underserved areas often miss out on early detection, leading to later-stage diagnoses and worse outcomes.

### The High Cost of Cancer Care

Cancer treatment in Western societies is notoriously expensive. The U.S. has some of the highest cancer treatment costs globally, with patients often facing financial ruin due to medical bills. While countries with universal healthcare, like Canada and much of Europe, provide more equitable access, disparities still exist in the quality and timeliness of care.

## Western vs. Non-Western Perspectives on Cancer

### Preventive Health in Non-Western Societies

Non-Western societies often take a more preventive approach to cancer. For example:
- Traditional Chinese Medicine (TCM) emphasizes balance in the body and incorporates herbal treatments that may reduce cancer risk.
- In India, turmeric—a key ingredient in many traditional dishes—contains curcumin, a compound studied for its anti-cancer properties.

### Cultural Attitudes Toward Cancer

Cultural attitudes also influence how cancer is perceived and treated. In Western societies, cancer is often framed as a battle, with patients seen as warriors. In contrast, some non-Western cultures emphasize acceptance and holistic healing.

### Cancer Disparities Within the West

Race and Ethnicity

Cancer outcomes vary significantly among racial and ethnic groups in Western societies. For example:
- African Americans in the U.S. have higher death rates from most cancers than any other racial group, often due to delayed diagnoses and unequal access to care.
- Hispanic and Asian populations tend to have lower cancer rates overall but face unique risks, such as higher rates of stomach cancer in Asian communities due to dietary factors.

Socioeconomic Status

Income inequality is another major driver of cancer disparities. Lower-income individuals are less likely to have access to preventive care, nutritious food, and timely treatment, contributing to higher mortality rates.

Conclusion: Cancer as a Reflection of Society

Cancer in Western society is a multifaceted issue shaped by lifestyle, environment, and healthcare systems. It highlights the paradox of modern living: the same advances that have extended life expectancy and improved quality of life have also introduced new risks. By examining these factors, we can better understand how to prevent and treat cancer in the context of our rapidly changing world.

## Chapter 4: The Business of Cancer

Cancer is not just a devastating disease—it is a multibillion-dollar industry. From diagnostics and pharmaceuticals to fundraising campaigns and advocacy groups, the economic ecosystem surrounding cancer is vast and complex. While this industry has led to life-saving advancements, it also raises critical questions about ethics, accessibility, and whether the financial incentives align with finding a cure.

### The Cancer Economy: A Snapshot

Globally, cancer care is estimated to be a $200 billion industry, and it's growing every year. In the United States alone, cancer costs reached over $200 billion in 2020, encompassing medical treatments, hospitalizations, diagnostic testing, and out-of-pocket expenses for patients. The pharmaceutical sector plays a significant role, with some single cancer drugs generating billions in revenue annually.

Breakdown of the Cancer Industry
- Diagnostics: Imaging tests (CT, MRI, PET scans), biopsies, and genetic testing.
- Treatments: Chemotherapy, radiation therapy, immunotherapy, and surgical procedures.
- Pharmaceuticals: Anti-cancer drugs, targeted therapies, and supportive care medications (e.g., anti-nausea drugs).
- Support Services: Palliative care, counseling, and rehabilitation services.
- Advocacy and Fundraising: Non-profits and charities like the American Cancer Society and Stand Up to Cancer.

The sheer scale of this industry highlights its importance in saving lives, but it also reveals the financial stakes that drive decision-making in cancer research and care.

The Profit Motive: Help or Hindrance?

Pharmaceutical Giants and Drug Pricing

One of the most controversial aspects of the cancer industry is the pricing of cancer drugs. Some medications cost over $100,000 per year, placing them out of reach for many patients, even in wealthy countries. For example:

- Immunotherapy Drugs: Treatments like pembrolizumab (Keytruda) are revolutionary but come with staggering price tags.
- Targeted Therapies: Drugs like imatinib (Gleevec), which target specific genetic mutations, initially launched at $26,000 per year but have since soared to over $120,000 annually.

Pharmaceutical companies argue that high prices are necessary to fund research and development. However, critics point out that much of the foundational research for these drugs is publicly funded, and companies often prioritize profit over accessibility.

The Patent System

Patents give pharmaceutical companies exclusive rights to market new drugs, often for 20 years or more. This monopoly allows them to set high prices, limiting access in low- and middle-income countries. The system also discourages competition, delaying the availability of cheaper generic alternatives.

## Non-Profits and Fundraising: Where Does the Money Go?

Cancer charities play a vital role in funding research, raising awareness, and supporting patients. Organizations like the American Cancer Society, Susan G. Komen Foundation, and Cancer Research UK have raised billions of dollars. However, their effectiveness has been questioned.

### Administrative Costs and Transparency

A significant portion of donations to large charities often goes toward administrative expenses, marketing, and salaries, leaving less for research or patient support. Critics argue that some organizations prioritize fundraising over tangible results.

### Success Stories

Despite these criticisms, many non-profits have made meaningful contributions to cancer research. For example, the Leukemia & Lymphoma Society funded early trials of

CAR-T therapy, a groundbreaking treatment for blood cancers.

## Clinical Trials: A Double-Edged Sword

Clinical trials are essential for advancing cancer treatment, but they also raise ethical and economic questions.

### Access and Equity

Participation in clinical trials often depends on geographic location, income level, and healthcare access. Many trials are conducted in urban centers, excluding rural and underserved populations.

### The Financial Burden on Patients

While trials offer access to cutting-edge treatments, they often involve significant out-of-pocket costs, such as travel and lodging. In the U.S., only 5% of adult cancer patients participate in clinical trials, partly due to these barriers.

## The Role of Health Insurance

In Western countries like the United States, health insurance often dictates a patient's ability to access timely and comprehensive cancer care. Even with insurance, patients frequently face high deductibles, co-pays, and out-of-pocket expenses.

Financial Toxicity

The term "financial toxicity" describes the economic burden cancer patients endure. A study by the American Journal of Medicine found that 42% of cancer patients deplete their life savings within two years of diagnosis. Financial stress has been linked to worse treatment outcomes, creating a vicious cycle.

Contrast with Universal Healthcare

Countries with universal healthcare systems, such as Canada, the UK, and many in Europe, generally provide more equitable access to cancer care. However, these systems are not without challenges, including long wait times and limited access to the newest treatments.

Is a Cure Possible—or Profitable?

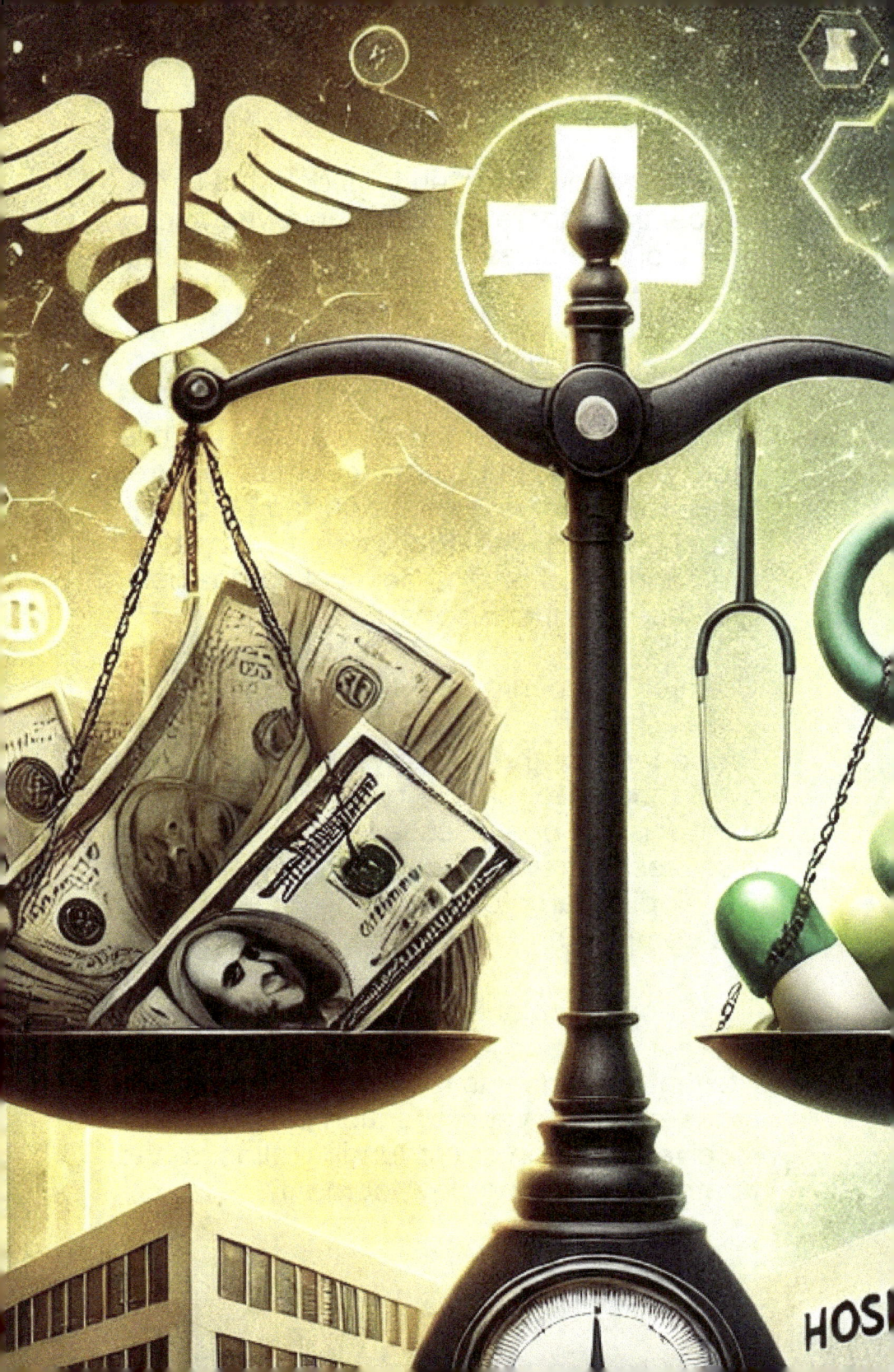

One of the most contentious debates in the cancer industry revolves around whether financial incentives hinder the development of a cure.

## The Conspiracy Theory

Critics of the cancer industry argue that it is more profitable to treat cancer than to cure it. While this theory is not supported by hard evidence, it reflects public skepticism about the priorities of pharmaceutical companies and research institutions.

## Counterarguments

Proponents of the industry argue that no single "cure" for cancer exists because cancer is not one disease but a collection of diseases with unique characteristics. Developing targeted therapies for each type is a complex and resource-intensive process.

## The Economics of Prevention

Preventing cancer is far more cost-effective than treating it, yet prevention programs receive a fraction of the funding allocated to treatment and drug development.

Underfunded Prevention Efforts
- Vaccination programs (e.g., HPV, Hepatitis B) are underutilized in many regions, despite their proven effectiveness.
- Public health campaigns to reduce smoking, improve diets, and encourage physical activity often face budget cuts.

The Role of Governments and NGOs

Governments and non-profits have stepped in to fill the gap, launching initiatives like anti-smoking campaigns and screening programs. However, these efforts need more robust funding and global coordination to reach their full potential.

Patient Advocacy and Grassroots Movements

Patients and survivors have become powerful advocates for change in the cancer industry. Grassroots movements and online communities have given patients a platform to share their stories, demand affordable treatments, and push for policy reforms.

Notable Movements

- Pink Ribbon Campaigns: Advocacy for breast cancer awareness has led to increased funding and public support for research.
- Right to Try Laws: These laws allow terminally ill patients to access experimental treatments outside clinical trials, sparking debates about safety and equity.

## Conclusion: The Dual Nature of the Cancer Industry

The cancer industry is both a source of hope and a target of criticism. It has driven remarkable progress in research and treatment, saving millions of lives. At the same time, its profit-driven model raises ethical questions about accessibility and equity.

As we continue to invest in cancer care, it is essential to prioritize not just innovation but also affordability, prevention, and global collaboration. Only then can we ensure that the fight against cancer truly serves humanity.

## Part IV: The Cancers A-Z Directory

This section is the heart of *Cancer-Us*, an exhaustive directory of all known cancers, categorized alphabetically. For each cancer, we provide an in-depth exploration, including definitions, history, causes, treatments, prevention strategies, and global perspectives. Let's begin with a detailed draft for the A section.

# A

## 1. Acute Lymphoblastic Leukemia (ALL)

**Definition:**
Acute Lymphoblastic Leukemia (ALL) is a type of blood cancer characterized by the overproduction of immature lymphocytes (a type of white blood cell) in the bone marrow. It is most common in children but can also occur in adults.

**History:**
- First described in the 19th century as a "white blood disease."
- Major advances in chemotherapy during the mid-20th century revolutionized treatment, leading to high cure rates in children.

**Causes:**
- Genetic mutations in lymphoid cells.
- Risk factors include exposure to radiation, certain chemicals, and genetic disorders like Down syndrome.

**Symptoms:**
- Fatigue, fever, frequent infections.
- Bruising, bleeding, and bone or joint pain.

**Treatments:**
- Medical: Combination chemotherapy (induction, consolidation, and maintenance phases), bone marrow transplants, targeted therapies (e.g., blinatumomab).
- Natural/Supportive: Dietary changes to support the immune system, stress-reducing practices like yoga and meditation.

**Prevention:**
- Currently no known prevention, but early detection improves outcomes.

**Global Perspective:**

- In high-income countries, childhood ALL has a survival rate exceeding 90%.
- In low-income countries, limited access to treatment reduces survival rates to below 50%.

Personal Story:
Emily, diagnosed at age 6, underwent two years of chemotherapy. Now cancer-free, she advocates for early detection programs in underserved communities.

## 2. Acute Myeloid Leukemia (AML)

Definition:
Acute Myeloid Leukemia (AML) is an aggressive cancer that affects the myeloid line of blood cells, leading to the rapid accumulation of immature blood cells in the bone marrow.

History:
- Identified in the late 19th century through advancements in blood microscopy.
- Modern treatment options emerged in the mid-20th century.

Causes:

- Genetic mutations in bone marrow cells.
- Risk factors: exposure to benzene, smoking, prior chemotherapy, and genetic conditions like Fanconi anemia.

Symptoms:
- Fatigue, weight loss, easy bruising.
- Recurrent infections and pale skin.

Treatments:
- Medical: Induction chemotherapy (e.g., cytarabine, daunorubicin), stem cell transplantation, targeted therapies like midostaurin.
- Natural/Supportive: Nutritional support to maintain strength during treatment, acupuncture for nausea relief.

Prevention:
- Avoidance of known carcinogens like benzene.
- Smoking cessation programs.

Global Perspective:
- Higher survival rates in countries with advanced healthcare infrastructure.

- Emerging research in India focuses on Ayurvedic herbs to complement traditional treatments.

Personal Story:
James, a 45-year-old firefighter, developed AML after years of exposure to smoke and chemicals. Following a stem cell transplant, he has been in remission for five years.

## 3. Adrenal Cancer

Definition:
Adrenal cancer is a rare cancer that begins in the adrenal glands, which produce hormones like adrenaline and cortisol.

History:
- First described in medical literature in the 19th century.
- Remains rare, with fewer than 2 cases per million people annually.

Causes:
- Genetic mutations, often linked to syndromes like Li-Fraumeni or Lynch syndrome.
- Prolonged exposure to certain environmental toxins may play a role.

Symptoms:
- Hormonal imbalances: high blood pressure, weight gain, or unexplained fatigue.
- Pain or a lump in the abdominal area.

Treatments:
- Medical: Surgical removal of the adrenal gland, chemotherapy (mitotane), and radiation therapy.
- Natural/Supportive: Hormone-regulating diets, mindfulness practices to reduce stress.

Prevention:
- Genetic counseling for individuals with a family history of adrenal cancer.
- Regular screenings for high-risk individuals.

Global Perspective:
- Limited data due to the rarity of the disease, but advanced treatment centers in the U.S. and Europe have improved outcomes.

Personal Story:
Sofia, diagnosed at age 30 during a routine health check, underwent successful surgery

and now raises awareness about the importance of early detection.

## 4. Anal Cancer

**Definition:**
Anal cancer develops in the tissues of the anus, often associated with human papillomavirus (HPV) infection.

**History:**
- Historically considered rare, but rates have been increasing due to the prevalence of HPV.
- Advances in the HPV vaccine have helped reduce risk.

**Causes:**
- HPV infection is the most significant risk factor.
- Smoking, anal intercourse, and immunosuppression also contribute.

**Symptoms:**
- Rectal bleeding, pain or itching in the anal area, and changes in bowel habits.

**Treatments:**

- Medical: Chemoradiation (5-fluorouracil and mitomycin), surgery for advanced cases.
- Natural/Supportive: High-fiber diets to ease bowel movements, pelvic floor exercises to reduce discomfort.

Prevention:
- HPV vaccination and safe sexual practices.
- Smoking cessation.

Global Perspective:
- In Western countries, HPV vaccination programs have significantly reduced rates of anal cancer.
- In low-income countries, lack of access to vaccines and screening contributes to higher mortality rates.

Personal Story:
Carlos, a 60-year-old, shared his experience with anal cancer in a local support group, highlighting the importance of early treatment and community support.

Part IV: The Cancers A-Z Directory

Continued: A

## 5. Appendiceal Cancer

**Definition:**
Appendiceal cancer is a rare type of cancer that starts in the appendix, a small organ attached to the large intestine. It often presents as a mucinous or non-mucinous adenocarcinoma or as carcinoid tumors.

**History:**
- First identified as a distinct cancer type in the early 20th century.
- Due to its rarity, research into appendiceal cancer has been slow to advance.

**Causes:**
- Exact causes are unknown. Genetic mutations are suspected to play a role.
- Risk factors include chronic appendicitis and hereditary cancer syndromes like Lynch syndrome.

**Symptoms:**
- Abdominal pain, bloating, or a mass in the abdomen.

- Symptoms may mimic appendicitis or remain asymptomatic until advanced stages.

Treatments:
- Medical: Surgery (appendectomy or cytoreductive surgery) combined with Hyperthermic Intraperitoneal Chemotherapy (HIPEC).
- Natural/Supportive: Anti-inflammatory diets and complementary therapies to manage post-surgical recovery.

Prevention:
- No known prevention methods due to its rarity, but routine monitoring for those with familial cancer syndromes is recommended.

Global Perspective:
- Advanced treatment centers in Europe and the U.S. specialize in HIPEC, improving survival rates for advanced cases.
- Limited treatment options in developing countries often lead to poorer outcomes.

Personal Story:
Beth, a 52-year-old teacher, was diagnosed with appendiceal cancer after routine surgery

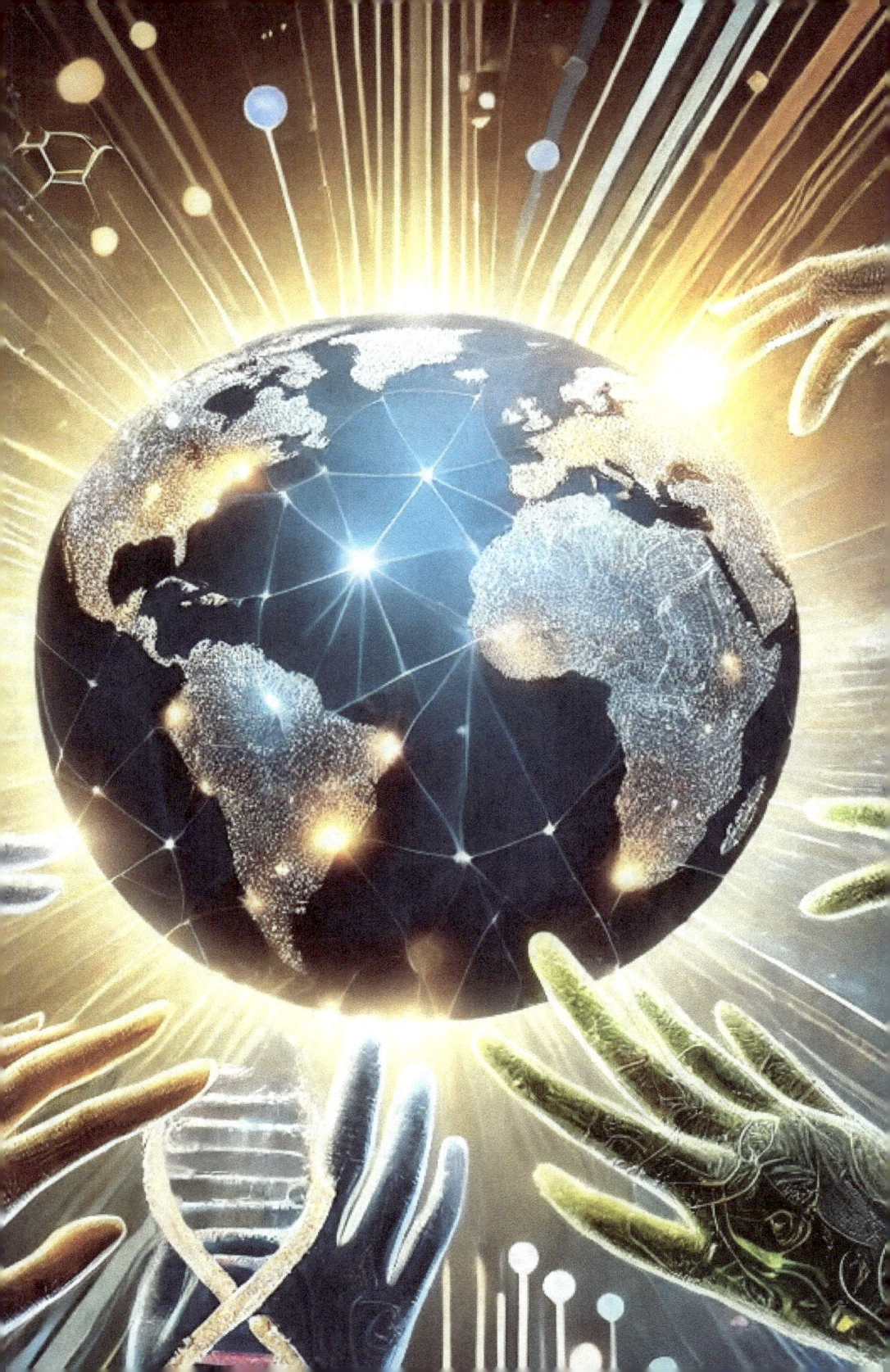

for what was thought to be appendicitis. Her participation in a clinical trial for HIPEC treatment gave her a new lease on life.

## 6. Astrocytoma

Definition:
Astrocytomas are tumors that arise from astrocytes, a type of glial cell in the brain and spinal cord. They can range from low-grade (slow-growing) to high-grade (aggressive, such as glioblastomas).

History:
- First classified as a distinct type of brain tumor in the 19th century.
- Advances in imaging technology have improved diagnosis over the past century.

Causes:
- Mutations in genes like IDH1 and TP53 are common.
- Risk factors include prior radiation exposure and inherited syndromes like Li-Fraumeni.

Symptoms:

- Seizures, headaches, and neurological deficits (e.g., vision changes, weakness).
- Cognitive or personality changes may occur in advanced stages.

Treatments:
- Medical: Surgery, radiation therapy, and chemotherapy (e.g., temozolomide). For high-grade astrocytomas, newer treatments like tumor-treating fields are being explored.
- Natural/Supportive: Diets emphasizing brain health (e.g., omega-3 fatty acids), mindfulness practices, and physical therapy.

Prevention:
- While most cases are sporadic, individuals with hereditary cancer syndromes should undergo regular screenings.

Global Perspective:
- Access to advanced imaging and treatment significantly affects outcomes.

Survival rates for high-grade astrocytomas are much higher in high-income countries.

Personal Story:
Liam, a 10-year-old boy diagnosed with a low-grade astrocytoma, underwent surgery and radiation therapy. His journey inspired a community fundraiser that brought awareness to pediatric brain cancer.

## 7. Asbestos-Related Cancers

Definition:
Cancers caused by asbestos exposure include mesothelioma (affecting the lining of the lungs, abdomen, or heart) and lung cancer. Asbestos fibers, when inhaled, can remain in the body for decades, causing cellular damage and cancer.

History:
- Linked to cancer in the early 20th century, asbestos was widely used in construction and manufacturing before its risks were recognized.
- Many countries banned asbestos in the late 20th century, but its effects persist.

Causes:
- Direct inhalation of asbestos fibers is the primary cause.
- Occupational exposure in construction, shipbuilding, and mining is most common.

Symptoms:
- Shortness of breath, persistent cough, and chest pain for mesothelioma.
- General lung cancer symptoms like coughing up blood and unexplained weight loss.

Treatments:
- Medical: Surgery (pleurectomy or extrapleural pneumonectomy), chemotherapy (pemetrexed and cisplatin), and radiation therapy.
- Natural/Supportive: Breathing exercises and anti-inflammatory diets to manage symptoms.

Prevention:
- Avoidance of asbestos exposure through regulation and protective gear.
- Regular health screenings for at-risk workers.

Global Perspective:

- Developed nations have largely banned asbestos, but it remains in use in many low- and middle-income countries, perpetuating its cancer risks.

Personal Story:
Henry, a retired shipbuilder, developed mesothelioma decades after exposure to asbestos. His legal battle for compensation brought attention to asbestos-related cancers and workplace safety.

8. Atypical Teratoid Rhabdoid Tumor (ATRT)

Definition:
ATRT is a rare, aggressive brain tumor that primarily affects children under the age of 3. It arises in the cerebellum or brainstem.

History:
- First identified in the 1980s.
- Research into its genetic underpinnings began in the late 1990s, linking it to mutations in the SMARCB1 gene.

Causes:
- Mutations in the SMARCB1 gene, often without hereditary links.

Symptoms:
- Nausea, vomiting, lethargy, and difficulty with balance or coordination.

Treatments:
- Medical: Surgery, intensive chemotherapy, and radiation therapy. Newer approaches include proton therapy to minimize damage to healthy tissues.
- Natural/Supportive: Nutritional support for young patients undergoing aggressive treatment.

Prevention:
- No known prevention due to its genetic nature.

Global Perspective:
- Access to pediatric oncology expertise is critical but limited in many parts of the world.

Personal Story:
Mia, diagnosed at 18 months, underwent a combination of surgery and chemotherapy. Her family's advocacy has raised over $1 million for pediatric cancer research.

Part IV: The Cancers A-Z Directory

Continued: B

1. Basal Cell Carcinoma (BCC)

Definition:
Basal Cell Carcinoma (BCC) is the most common form of skin cancer. It arises from the basal cells in the epidermis, typically due to prolonged sun exposure. Though rarely fatal, BCC can cause significant disfigurement if untreated.

History:
- First formally identified in the 19th century by pathologists studying skin lesions.
- Advances in dermatology and early detection programs have made it one of the most successfully treated cancers.

Causes:
- Chronic exposure to ultraviolet (UV) radiation from the sun or tanning beds.
- Fair skin, a history of sunburns, and immunosuppression increase risk.

Symptoms:
- A pearly, flesh-colored bump or a pink patch of skin, often on the face or neck.

- Lesions may bleed, crust, or develop a central depression over time.

Treatments:
- Medical: Mohs surgery, topical treatments like imiquimod, cryotherapy, and in advanced cases, targeted drugs like vismodegib.
- Natural/Supportive: Protective clothing and sunscreen to prevent recurrence. Some patients use aloe vera and vitamin C creams to soothe affected skin.

Prevention:
- Consistent use of sunscreen and protective clothing.
- Regular skin checks, especially for individuals with a history of sun exposure.

Global Perspective:
- Higher rates in regions with intense sunlight, such as Australia and Southern U.S. states.
- Public health campaigns in these areas emphasize UV protection.

Personal Story:
Jack, an avid surfer from California, developed BCC on his nose. After Mohs surgery, he became a vocal advocate for skin

cancer awareness, encouraging young people to protect their skin.

## 2. Bile Duct Cancer (Cholangiocarcinoma)

Definition:
Bile duct cancer originates in the bile ducts, which carry bile from the liver to the gallbladder and small intestine. It is rare but aggressive, often diagnosed at advanced stages.

History:
- First classified in the early 20th century.
- Recent advancements in imaging technology have improved early detection.

Causes:
- Chronic liver diseases such as primary sclerosing cholangitis.
- Parasitic infections like liver flukes (common in Southeast Asia).
- Genetic mutations and bile duct inflammation.

Symptoms:

- Jaundice (yellowing of the skin and eyes), abdominal pain, unexplained weight loss, and dark urine.

Treatments:
- Medical: Surgery (bile duct resection or liver transplant), chemotherapy, and radiation. Targeted therapies like FGFR inhibitors are emerging options.
- Natural/Supportive: Milk thistle and turmeric are sometimes used for liver support, though evidence is limited.

Prevention:
- Avoiding parasitic infections by consuming properly cooked fish in endemic regions.
- Managing liver diseases and avoiding excessive alcohol consumption.

Global Perspective:
- High rates in Southeast Asia due to liver fluke infections. Efforts in these regions focus on eradicating parasites and increasing awareness of the risks.

Personal Story:
Vinh, a farmer from Vietnam, was diagnosed with bile duct cancer linked to liver flukes. Despite limited resources, a community

fundraiser helped him access surgery, extending his life significantly.

## 3. Bladder Cancer

**Definition:**
Bladder cancer begins in the cells lining the bladder. It is one of the most common urological cancers, particularly in older adults.

**History:**
- Documented as early as the 18th century when occupational exposure to dyes was linked to bladder cancer.
- Modern treatments emerged in the mid-20th century with the advent of chemotherapy and immunotherapy.

**Causes:**
- Smoking is the leading cause, accounting for approximately half of all cases.
- Occupational exposure to carcinogens such as aromatic amines in the dye and chemical industries.
- Chronic bladder inflammation and infections.

**Symptoms:**

- Blood in the urine (hematuria), frequent urination, and pelvic pain.

Treatments:
- Medical: Transurethral resection of bladder tumors (TURBT), intravesical therapy (e.g., BCG immunotherapy), and systemic chemotherapy for advanced cases.
- Natural/Supportive: Hydration and diets rich in antioxidants may support bladder health.

Prevention:
- Smoking cessation and avoidance of chemical exposure.
- Early treatment of urinary tract infections and other bladder conditions.

Global Perspective:
- Higher rates in industrialized nations due to occupational risks and smoking prevalence.
- In parts of Africa and the Middle East, bladder cancer is often linked to schistosomiasis, a parasitic infection.

Personal Story:
Margaret, a retired chemist, developed bladder cancer linked to her work in dye manufacturing. Her journey through TURBT

and immunotherapy inspired her to advocate for stricter workplace safety regulations.

## 4. Brain Cancer (Glioblastoma and Other Types)

Definition:
Brain cancer includes various tumors originating in the brain. Glioblastoma, the most aggressive type, accounts for 15% of all brain tumors.

History:
- Brain tumors were first documented in ancient Egyptian texts.
- The development of modern imaging techniques revolutionized diagnosis in the 20th century.

Causes:
- Genetic mutations and hereditary syndromes like Li-Fraumeni.
- Environmental exposures to radiation or industrial chemicals.
- The exact causes of many brain cancers remain unknown.

Symptoms:

- Persistent headaches, seizures, cognitive impairments, and personality changes.
- Motor function difficulties and vision problems.

Treatments:
- Medical: Surgery, radiation therapy, and chemotherapy (e.g., temozolomide for glioblastoma). Emerging treatments include tumor-treating fields and immunotherapy.
- Natural/Supportive: Omega-3-rich diets, mindfulness practices, and physical therapy to support recovery.

Prevention:
- Limited options due to the unknown etiology of many brain tumors.
- Reducing radiation exposure and managing hereditary risks may help.

Global Perspective:
- Access to advanced neurosurgical centers significantly improves survival rates in developed countries.
- In low-income regions, delayed diagnosis often leads to poorer outcomes.

Personal Story:

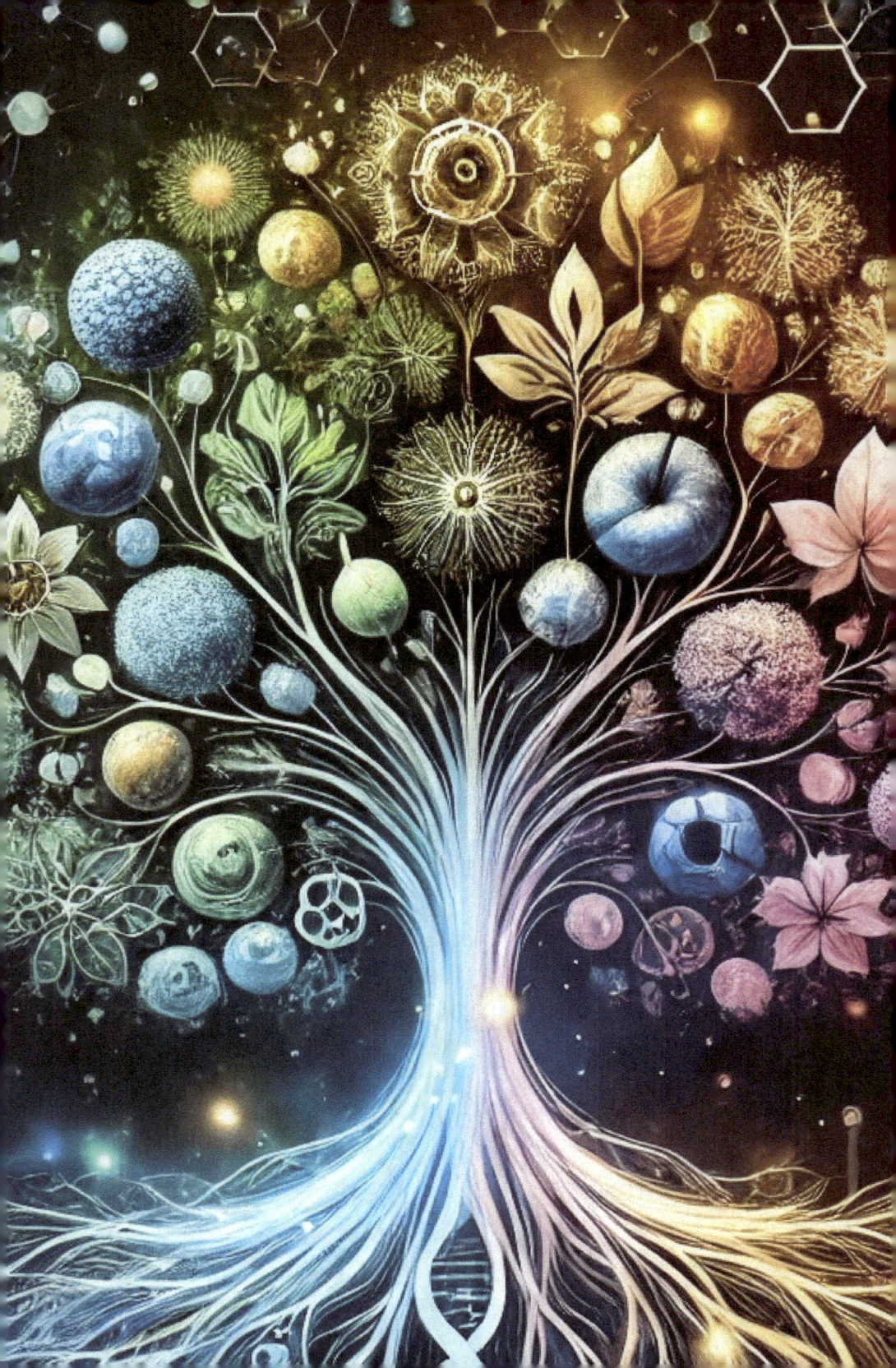

Sarah, a 34-year-old teacher, was diagnosed with glioblastoma after persistent headaches. Her fight inspired her community to fundraise for cutting-edge treatments, including a clinical trial for immunotherapy.

## 5. Breast Cancer

Definition:
Breast cancer arises in the cells of the breast, most commonly in the ducts or lobules. It is the most common cancer in women worldwide, though men can also develop it.

History:
- Mentioned in ancient Egyptian texts, with mastectomies performed as early as 500 BCE.
- Modern advancements, including mammography and targeted therapies, have revolutionized outcomes.

Causes:
- Genetic mutations like BRCA1 and BRCA2.
- Hormonal factors, obesity, alcohol consumption, and radiation exposure.

Symptoms:

- A lump in the breast, changes in breast shape, nipple discharge, or skin dimpling.

Treatments:
- Medical: Surgery (lumpectomy or mastectomy), chemotherapy, radiation, hormonal therapy (e.g., tamoxifen), and targeted drugs like trastuzumab.
- Natural/Supportive: Diets rich in cruciferous vegetables and mindfulness practices like yoga.

Prevention:
- Regular mammograms, self-exams, and lifestyle changes like maintaining a healthy weight.
- Preventive surgery for high-risk individuals (e.g., Angelina Jolie's mastectomy).

Global Perspective:
- High survival rates in developed nations due to early detection and advanced treatments.
- In developing countries, cultural stigmas and limited access to care delay diagnosis.

Personal Story:

Monica, a 55-year-old mother of three, credits her early diagnosis during a routine mammogram for saving her life. She now volunteers to educate underserved communities about breast cancer awareness.

## Part IV: The Cancers A-Z Directory

Continued: C

### 1. Cervical Cancer

**Definition:**
Cervical cancer develops in the cells lining the cervix, the lower part of the uterus connecting to the vagina. It is strongly associated with persistent infection by high-risk strains of the human papillomavirus (HPV).

**History:**
- Descriptions of cervical tumors date back to ancient Greece.
- In the 20th century, the Pap smear, developed by Dr. George Papanicolaou, revolutionized early detection.

**Causes:**

- HPV infection is the primary cause, particularly types 16 and 18.
- Other risk factors include smoking, long-term use of oral contraceptives, and a weakened immune system.

Symptoms:
- Early stages are often asymptomatic.
- Symptoms include abnormal vaginal bleeding, pelvic pain, and unusual discharge.

Treatments:
- Medical: Surgery (hysterectomy or cone biopsy), radiation therapy, and chemotherapy. Immunotherapy and targeted therapies are emerging options.
- Natural/Supportive: Anti-inflammatory diets and herbal supplements like green tea extract (studied for its potential antiviral properties).

Prevention:
- Routine Pap smears and HPV testing.
- Vaccination against HPV, recommended for adolescents.
- Safe sexual practices and smoking cessation.

Global Perspective:
- Developed nations have seen a dramatic decrease in cases due to vaccination and screening programs.
- In low-income countries, cervical cancer remains a leading cause of cancer death in women due to limited access to preventive care.

Personal Story:
Anika, a 32-year-old mother from India, was diagnosed with cervical cancer at an advanced stage. After treatment, she became an advocate for HPV vaccination in rural areas, helping hundreds of girls get vaccinated.

## 2. Colorectal Cancer

Definition:
Colorectal cancer affects the colon (large intestine) or rectum. It is one of the most common cancers worldwide, often developing from precancerous polyps.

History:
- Colorectal cancer has been documented in ancient medical texts.

- The introduction of colonoscopy in the mid-20th century revolutionized early detection.

Causes:
- Genetic mutations in the APC gene, Lynch syndrome, and familial adenomatous polyposis.
- Lifestyle factors, including diets high in red and processed meats, low fiber intake, obesity, and alcohol consumption.

Symptoms:
- Changes in bowel habits, rectal bleeding, abdominal pain, and unexplained weight loss.

Treatments:
- Medical: Surgery (polypectomy, colectomy), chemotherapy (e.g., FOLFOX), and radiation therapy. Targeted therapies like cetuximab for advanced cases.
- Natural/Supportive: High-fiber diets, probiotics for gut health, and regular exercise to improve recovery.

Prevention:
- Routine colonoscopies starting at age 45 or earlier for high-risk individuals.

- Diets rich in fruits, vegetables, and whole grains.

Global Perspective:
- High rates in Western countries, likely linked to dietary habits.
- Public health campaigns in Australia and the U.S. emphasize screening and lifestyle changes to reduce incidence.

Personal Story:
Tom, a 50-year-old engineer, was diagnosed during a routine colonoscopy. Early detection allowed for minimally invasive surgery, and he now advocates for routine screenings among his peers.

## 3. Cutaneous T-Cell Lymphoma (CTCL)

Definition:
Cutaneous T-cell lymphoma is a rare type of non-Hodgkin lymphoma that originates in the T-cells of the immune system and affects the skin.

History:
- First described in the 19th century, with subtypes like Mycosis Fungoides becoming better understood in the 20th century.

- Advances in immunotherapy have provided new treatment options.

Causes:
- The exact cause is unknown, but genetic mutations and immune system dysregulation are suspected.
- Risk factors include a history of autoimmune diseases and certain viral infections.

Symptoms:
- Red, scaly patches or plaques on the skin that can resemble eczema or psoriasis.
- Itching and, in advanced stages, tumor formation.

Treatments:
- Medical: Topical steroids, phototherapy, systemic therapies (e.g., bexarotene), and stem cell transplants for advanced cases.
- Natural/Supportive: Moisturizing ointments and anti-inflammatory diets to reduce skin irritation.

Prevention:

- No established prevention due to the rarity and unknown causes of the disease.

Global Perspective:
- More common in older adults and slightly more prevalent in men.
- Advanced treatments are primarily available in high-income countries.

Personal Story:
Denise, a 68-year-old retired teacher, struggled with CTCL misdiagnosis for years. Access to a specialist finally provided clarity, and she now volunteers to raise awareness about rare cancers.

## 4. Chondrosarcoma

Definition:
Chondrosarcoma is a type of bone cancer that arises in cartilage cells. It is most common in adults and usually affects the pelvis, femur, or ribs.

History:
- Identified in the early 20th century as a distinct type of sarcoma.
- Advances in imaging techniques have improved early detection.

**Causes:**
- Genetic mutations in the IDH1 or COL2A1 genes.
- Risk factors include pre-existing conditions like Ollier disease or Maffucci syndrome.

**Symptoms:**
- Persistent pain in the affected bone, swelling, and reduced range of motion.

**Treatments:**
- Medical: Surgery is the primary treatment, as chondrosarcomas are resistant to chemotherapy and radiation. Advanced cases may require limb-sparing techniques or amputation.
- Natural/Supportive: Physical therapy and pain management strategies.

**Prevention:**
- Regular monitoring for individuals with genetic predispositions.

**Global Perspective:**
- Most cases occur sporadically, with no major geographic disparities.
- Access to specialized orthopedic oncologists is critical for effective treatment.

**Personal Story:**
Luca, a 35-year-old athlete, underwent limb-sparing surgery for chondrosarcoma. His experience led him to establish a foundation supporting young adults facing bone cancer.

## Part IV: The Cancers A-Z Directory

**Continued: C**

### 5. Chronic Lymphocytic Leukemia (CLL)

**Definition:**
Chronic Lymphocytic Leukemia (CLL) is a slow-growing blood cancer that affects lymphocytes, a type of white blood cell. It is most common in older adults and often detected during routine blood tests.

**History:**
- First recognized as a distinct type of leukemia in the mid-19th century.
- Advances in targeted therapies over the last two decades have significantly improved outcomes.

**Causes:**
- Genetic mutations in lymphoid cells.

- Risk factors include a family history of leukemia and exposure to certain chemicals like Agent Orange.

Symptoms:
- Fatigue, swollen lymph nodes, frequent infections, and night sweats.
- Often asymptomatic in early stages.

Treatments:
- Medical: Watchful waiting for early-stage cases, targeted therapies (e.g., ibrutinib), monoclonal antibodies, and chemotherapy.
- Natural/Supportive: Diets rich in antioxidants, stress management, and exercise to boost immune function.

Prevention:
- No definitive prevention, but avoiding known carcinogens and maintaining overall health may reduce risk.

Global Perspective:
- Higher rates in Western countries compared to Asia and Africa, possibly due to genetic and environmental factors.
- Advanced therapies are more accessible in developed nations.

Personal Story:
Richard, a 68-year-old retired teacher, managed his CLL with a combination of targeted therapy and lifestyle changes, allowing him to maintain an active lifestyle and advocate for cancer awareness in his community.

## 6. Chronic Myeloid Leukemia (CML)

Definition:
Chronic Myeloid Leukemia (CML) is a blood cancer characterized by the overproduction of abnormal white blood cells due to a genetic mutation called the Philadelphia chromosome.

History:
- First described in the mid-19th century, the discovery of the Philadelphia chromosome in 1960 was a major breakthrough in cancer research.
- The development of imatinib (Gleevec) in the early 2000s transformed CML from a fatal disease to a manageable condition.

Causes:

- The Philadelphia chromosome, resulting from a translocation between chromosomes 9 and 22.
- No clear environmental or hereditary risk factors.

Symptoms:
- Fatigue, night sweats, fever, and an enlarged spleen.

Treatments:
- Medical: Tyrosine kinase inhibitors (e.g., imatinib, dasatinib), chemotherapy, and bone marrow transplants for advanced cases.
- Natural/Supportive: Nutritional support during treatment, yoga, and mindfulness for stress reduction.

Prevention:
- No known prevention methods due to its genetic origin.

Global Perspective:
- Access to tyrosine kinase inhibitors has dramatically improved survival rates in developed countries.
- High costs limit availability in low-income regions.

Personal Story:
Anne, a 45-year-old graphic designer, credits imatinib for allowing her to lead a normal life despite her CML diagnosis. She now mentors newly diagnosed patients to help them navigate treatment.

## 7. Colon Cancer

Definition:
Colon cancer originates in the large intestine and is one of the most common cancers globally. It often develops from precancerous polyps that gradually become malignant.

History:
- Documented in medical literature as early as the 17th century.
- Screening methods like colonoscopy, developed in the 20th century, have significantly reduced mortality rates.

Causes:
- Genetic mutations, such as in the APC or KRAS genes.
- Lifestyle factors: diets high in red meat, low fiber intake, obesity, smoking, and alcohol consumption.

**Symptoms:**
- Changes in bowel habits, blood in the stool, abdominal discomfort, and unexplained weight loss.

**Treatments:**
- Medical: Surgery (polypectomy, colectomy), chemotherapy, radiation, and targeted therapies (e.g., bevacizumab).
- Natural/Supportive: High-fiber diets, probiotics for gut health, and physical activity to improve recovery.

**Prevention:**
- Routine colonoscopies starting at age 45.
- Diets rich in fruits, vegetables, and whole grains.
- Avoiding smoking and excessive alcohol consumption.

**Global Perspective:**
- High rates in Western countries due to dietary and lifestyle factors.
- Public health campaigns in countries like Australia and the U.S. emphasize early screening and healthy eating.

Personal Story:
Tom, a 50-year-old engineer, underwent minimally invasive surgery after a routine colonoscopy detected early-stage colon cancer. He now encourages others to prioritize preventive health checks.

## 8. Conjunctival Melanoma

Definition:
Conjunctival melanoma is a rare type of eye cancer that develops in the conjunctiva, the thin membrane covering the eye's surface.

History:
- First classified as a distinct melanoma subtype in the early 20th century.
- Advances in ocular oncology have improved early detection and treatment options.

Causes:
- Mutations in genes like BRAF and NRAS.
- Risk factors include excessive UV exposure and pre-existing conjunctival pigmentation.

Symptoms:

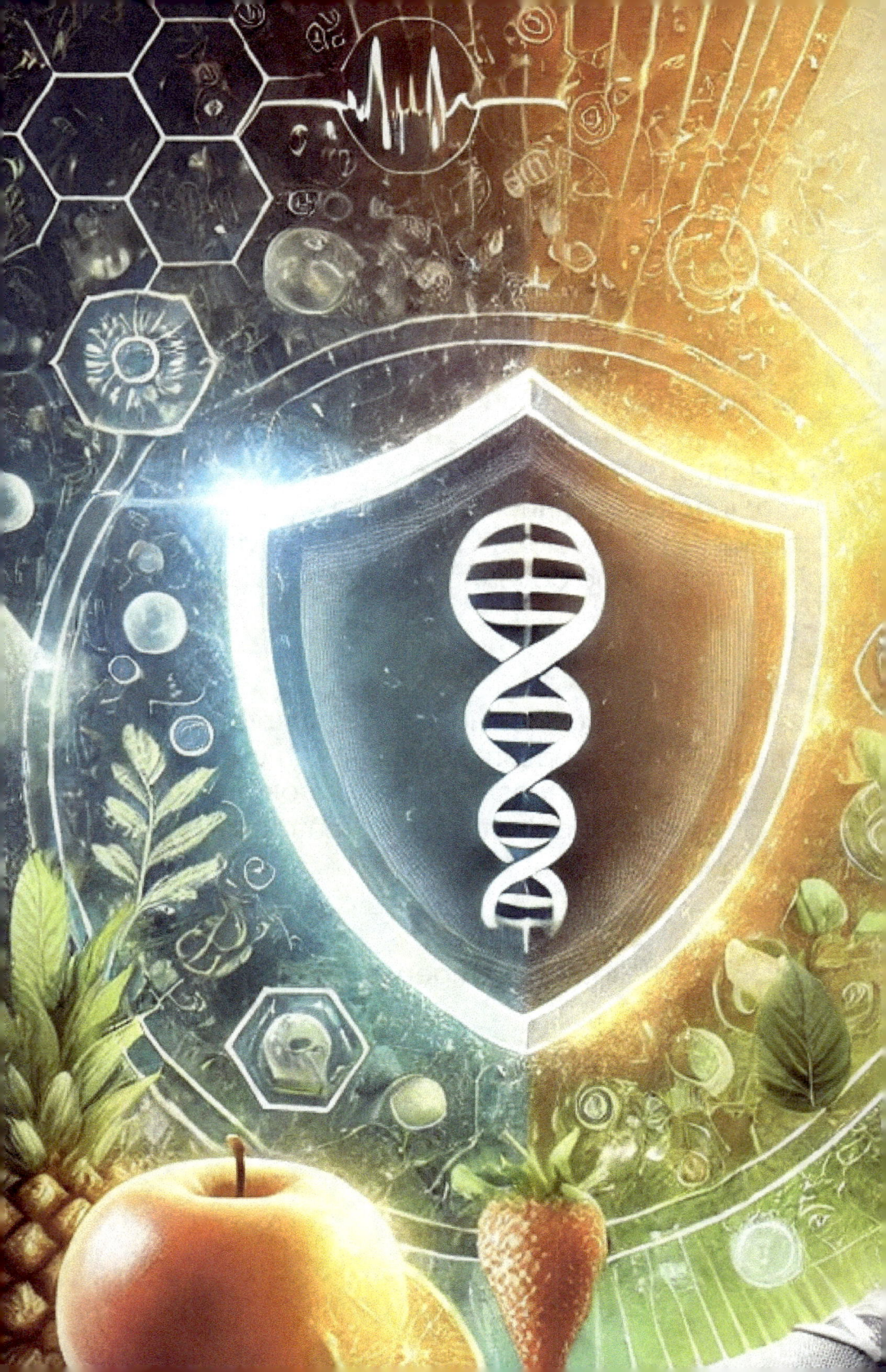

- A pigmented or non-pigmented lesion on the conjunctiva, often accompanied by irritation or redness.

Treatments:
- Medical: Surgical excision, cryotherapy, and radiation therapy. Targeted therapies and immunotherapy are under investigation.
- Natural/Supportive: Protective eyewear to reduce UV exposure and antioxidant-rich diets for eye health.

Prevention:
- Regular eye exams and UV protection.

Global Perspective:
- Higher incidence in fair-skinned individuals living in regions with high UV exposure.
- Access to specialized ocular oncologists is critical for effective treatment.

Personal Story:
Rachel, an avid hiker, discovered a lesion on her eye during a routine optometrist visit. Early intervention allowed her to avoid vision loss, and she now advocates for sun safety awareness.

## 9. Cardiac Sarcoma

**Definition:**
Cardiac sarcoma is a rare and aggressive cancer that originates in the heart's tissues, often in the left atrium.

**History:**
- First identified in the 19th century, cardiac sarcoma remains poorly understood due to its rarity.

**Causes:**
- Genetic mutations, though the exact triggers are largely unknown.
- Potential links to radiation exposure and previous cardiac surgeries.

**Symptoms:**
- Shortness of breath, chest pain, arrhythmias, and swelling in the legs.

**Treatments:**
- Medical: Surgery to remove the tumor, followed by chemotherapy or radiation therapy. Heart transplantation is considered in extreme cases.

- **Natural/Supportive:** Low-sodium diets and physical therapy to support cardiovascular health.

**Prevention:**
- No known prevention due to its sporadic occurrence.

**Global Perspective:**
- Access to advanced cardiac surgical teams is crucial but often limited to high-income countries.

**Personal Story:**
David, a 40-year-old marathon runner, was diagnosed with cardiac sarcoma after experiencing unexplained fatigue. His successful surgery inspired him to raise funds for rare cancer research.

## Part IV: The Cancers A-Z Directory

Continued: D

### 1. Desmoid Tumors (Aggressive Fibromatosis)

**Definition:**

Desmoid tumors are rare, non-metastatic soft tissue tumors that arise from connective tissue. Despite being non-cancerous, they can be aggressive, invading nearby structures and causing significant complications.

History:
- First described in the 19th century.
- Advances in genetic research have linked these tumors to mutations in the CTNNB1 gene or APC gene in familial cases.

Causes:
- Genetic mutations in connective tissue cells.
- Associated with Gardner's syndrome, a variant of familial adenomatous polyposis.

Symptoms:
- A firm, painless lump, often in the abdomen, shoulder, or thigh.
- Symptoms depend on the tumor's location and size, potentially causing pain or restricted movement.

Treatments:
- Medical: Surgery, radiation therapy, or systemic treatments such as

tyrosine kinase inhibitors (e.g., sorafenib) for unresectable cases.
- Natural/Supportive: Anti-inflammatory diets and physical therapy to manage symptoms.

Prevention:
- Genetic counseling and regular screenings for individuals with familial adenomatous polyposis.

Global Perspective:
- Desmoid tumors are treated primarily in specialized centers in high-income countries.
- Limited awareness and misdiagnosis are common in underserved regions.

Personal Story:
Lena, a 35-year-old artist, discovered a desmoid tumor in her abdomen during a routine check-up. Her treatment journey inspired her to create artwork highlighting the emotional impact of rare diseases.

## 2. Diffuse Large B-Cell Lymphoma (DLBCL)

Definition:

DLBCL is the most common type of non-Hodgkin lymphoma, characterized by fast-growing tumors originating in B-lymphocytes, a type of white blood cell.

History:
- First identified as a distinct lymphoma subtype in the 20th century.
- Advances in targeted therapy have significantly improved outcomes.

Causes:
- Genetic mutations in B-cells.
- Risk factors include age, weakened immune systems, and infections like Epstein-Barr virus (EBV).

Symptoms:
- Enlarged lymph nodes, night sweats, fever, and unexplained weight loss.

Treatments:
- Medical: Chemotherapy (R-CHOP regimen), monoclonal antibodies (e.g., rituximab), and stem cell transplants for relapsed cases.
- Natural/Supportive: Nutritional support and complementary therapies like acupuncture for symptom management.

Prevention:
- No definitive prevention, but managing underlying conditions (e.g., HIV) may reduce risk.

Global Perspective:
- Higher survival rates in regions with access to advanced therapies.
- In low-income countries, lack of access to rituximab and chemotherapy limits treatment success.

Personal Story:
John, a 65-year-old veteran, was diagnosed with DLBCL after persistent fatigue. His treatment with the R-CHOP regimen resulted in remission, and he now shares his story in support groups.

## 3. Ductal Carcinoma In Situ (DCIS)

Definition:
DCIS is a non-invasive breast cancer where abnormal cells are confined to the milk ducts. While not life-threatening, it can progress to invasive breast cancer if untreated.

History:

- Recognized in the mid-20th century with the advent of mammography.
- Advances in imaging have increased early detection rates.

Causes:
- Genetic mutations in breast duct cells.
- Risk factors include a family history of breast cancer, hormone replacement therapy, and late menopause.

Symptoms:
- Often asymptomatic, detected during routine mammograms.
- Occasionally, a lump or nipple discharge may occur.

Treatments:
- Medical: Lumpectomy or mastectomy, often combined with radiation therapy. Hormonal therapy (e.g., tamoxifen) is used for hormone receptor-positive cases.
- Natural/Supportive: Healthy diets, regular exercise, and stress management.

Prevention:
- Routine mammograms and genetic counseling for high-risk individuals.

- Lifestyle changes to reduce overall breast cancer risk.

Global Perspective:
- High survival rates in developed nations due to widespread screening programs.
- In low-income countries, lack of access to mammography leads to delayed detection.

Personal Story:
Samantha, a 48-year-old teacher, was diagnosed with DCIS during a routine screening. After a successful lumpectomy, she became a vocal advocate for breast cancer awareness.

## 4. Dermatofibrosarcoma Protuberans (DFSP)

Definition:
DFSP is a rare type of soft tissue sarcoma that begins in the dermis, the inner layer of the skin. It is slow-growing but has a high rate of recurrence if not fully removed.

History:
- First described in the early 20th century.

- Molecular research has identified a fusion of the COL1A1 and PDGFB genes as a cause.

Causes:
- Genetic rearrangements leading to overproduction of growth factors in skin cells.

Symptoms:
- A firm, reddish or purplish lump on the skin, often painless but prone to enlargement.

Treatments:
- Medical: Mohs micrographic surgery for precise removal, imatinib (targeted therapy) for advanced cases.
- Natural/Supportive: Topical treatments to manage irritation and scarring.

Prevention:
- No known prevention due to its sporadic occurrence.

Global Perspective:
- Advanced surgical techniques like Mohs are primarily available in developed nations.
- Limited awareness often leads to delayed diagnosis in underserved areas.

**Personal Story:**
Carlos, a 29-year-old photographer, noticed a lump on his shoulder that turned out to be DFSP. After successful Mohs surgery, he now educates others about rare skin cancers.

## 5. Double-Hit Lymphoma

**Definition:**
Double-hit lymphoma is a rare and aggressive type of B-cell lymphoma characterized by genetic rearrangements involving MYC and BCL2 and/or BCL6 genes.

**History:**
- Identified as a distinct entity in the early 21st century.
- Advances in genetic testing have improved diagnosis and treatment strategies.

**Causes:**
- Genetic mutations in B-cells.
- Often arises spontaneously, with no clear environmental or hereditary risk factors.

**Symptoms:**
- Rapidly growing lymph nodes, fever, night sweats, and significant weight loss.

Treatments:
- Medical: Intensive chemotherapy regimens (e.g., DA-EPOCH-R), stem cell transplantation, and emerging CAR-T cell therapy.
- Natural/Supportive: Nutritional support during treatment and mindfulness techniques for stress management.

Prevention:
- No known prevention due to its genetic basis.

Global Perspective:
- High mortality rates in regions without access to advanced therapies.
- Specialized treatment centers in developed nations significantly improve outcomes.

Personal Story:
David, a 45-year-old software engineer, underwent CAR-T cell therapy after traditional chemotherapy failed. His remarkable recovery inspired him to advocate for greater accessibility to cutting-edge treatments.

Part IV: The Cancers A-Z Directory

Continued: E

## 1. Esophageal Cancer

Definition:
Esophageal cancer develops in the tissues of the esophagus, the muscular tube connecting the throat to the stomach. The two main types are squamous cell carcinoma and adenocarcinoma.

History:
- First documented in ancient medical texts, with significant advances in surgical treatment occurring in the 20th century.
- The rise of gastroesophageal reflux disease (GERD) and obesity has led to an increase in adenocarcinoma cases in Western countries.

Causes:
- Risk factors include smoking, heavy alcohol use, GERD, Barrett's esophagus, and obesity.

- Chronic irritation of the esophageal lining can lead to cellular changes and cancer.

Symptoms:
- Difficulty swallowing (dysphagia), chest pain, unintentional weight loss, and persistent coughing.

Treatments:
- Medical: Surgery (esophagectomy), radiation therapy, chemotherapy, and targeted therapies like trastuzumab for HER2-positive cases.
- Natural/Supportive: Anti-inflammatory diets, small frequent meals to aid swallowing, and complementary therapies like acupuncture for symptom relief.

Prevention:
- Avoiding tobacco and excessive alcohol consumption.
- Managing GERD with diet, medication, and weight loss.

Global Perspective:
- Squamous cell carcinoma is more common in developing countries, linked to smoking and alcohol.

- Adenocarcinoma is prevalent in Western nations, associated with GERD and obesity.

Personal Story:
Hassan, a 54-year-old farmer from Iran, developed esophageal cancer due to lifelong use of tobacco. After undergoing surgery and radiation, he now educates others about the risks of smoking in his rural community.

## 2. Ewing Sarcoma

Definition:
Ewing sarcoma is a rare type of bone or soft tissue cancer most commonly affecting children and young adults. It often begins in the pelvis, legs, or ribs.

History:
- First described in 1921 by Dr. James Ewing.
- Advances in chemotherapy during the late 20th century significantly improved survival rates.

Causes:
- Genetic rearrangements in the EWSR1 gene, often without hereditary links.

- No definitive environmental or lifestyle risk factors.

Symptoms:
- Bone pain, swelling, and fractures.
- Fever, fatigue, and weight loss in advanced stages.

Treatments:
- Medical: Combination chemotherapy, surgery, and radiation therapy.
- Natural/Supportive: Nutritional support to aid recovery and physical therapy to regain mobility.

Prevention:
- No known prevention due to its genetic nature.

Global Perspective:
- More common in Caucasian populations and rare in African and Asian populations.
- Limited access to advanced treatments in low-income countries leads to poorer outcomes.

Personal Story:

Maya, a 12-year-old soccer player, was diagnosed with Ewing sarcoma in her leg. After surgery and chemotherapy, she returned to the field, inspiring her team and community with her resilience.

## 3. Endometrial Cancer

**Definition:**
Endometrial cancer arises in the lining of the uterus (endometrium) and is the most common gynecologic cancer in developed countries.

**History:**
- Descriptions of uterine tumors date back to ancient times, with significant advances in surgical treatment in the 20th century.
- Hormonal therapies became a key treatment option in the mid-20th century.

**Causes:**
- Risk factors include obesity, hormone replacement therapy, early menstruation, late menopause, and genetic syndromes like Lynch syndrome.

- High levels of estrogen relative to progesterone can stimulate abnormal cell growth.

Symptoms:
- Abnormal uterine bleeding, pelvic pain, and unusual vaginal discharge.

Treatments:
- Medical: Surgery (hysterectomy), radiation therapy, hormonal therapy, and chemotherapy for advanced stages.
- Natural/Supportive: Weight management, diets rich in whole foods, and stress-reducing practices like yoga.

Prevention:
- Maintaining a healthy weight, managing hormone replacement therapy under medical supervision, and regular gynecologic exams.

Global Perspective:
- Higher rates in Western countries, linked to obesity and longer lifespans.
- In developing countries, lack of access to early detection results in poorer outcomes.

Personal Story:

Emma, a 59-year-old nurse, detected her endometrial cancer early due to persistent spotting after menopause. Her successful treatment inspired her to advocate for awareness about postmenopausal bleeding.

## 4. Embryonal Carcinoma (Testicular Cancer Subtype)

**Definition:**
Embryonal carcinoma is a rare and aggressive type of testicular cancer, classified as a non-seminomatous germ cell tumor. It often affects young men aged 15-35.

**History:**
- First identified in the 20th century as a distinct subtype of testicular cancer.
- Advancements in chemotherapy, particularly cisplatin-based regimens, have greatly improved survival rates.

**Causes:**
- Risk factors include undescended testicles (cryptorchidism), family history, and genetic mutations.

Symptoms:
- A lump or swelling in the testicle, back pain, and abdominal discomfort in advanced stages.

Treatments:
- Medical: Surgery (orchiectomy), chemotherapy, and radiation therapy.
- Natural/Supportive: Nutritional support and physical activity to maintain overall health during treatment.

Prevention:
- Regular self-exams and monitoring of testicular health.

Global Perspective:
- Higher incidence in Western countries, with significantly improved survival rates due to advanced treatments.
- Cultural stigma in some regions delays diagnosis and treatment.

Personal Story:
Jake, a 24-year-old college student, caught his embryonal carcinoma early during a self-exam. After surgery and chemotherapy, he

started a campaign encouraging young men to prioritize testicular health.

## 5. Extramedullary Plasmacytoma

Definition:
Extramedullary plasmacytoma is a rare type of cancer involving plasma cells that form tumors outside the bone marrow, often in the head and neck region.

History:
- First recognized as a distinct condition in the mid-20th century.
- Advances in imaging and radiation therapy have improved diagnosis and outcomes.

Causes:
- Often linked to underlying conditions like multiple myeloma.
- Risk factors include chronic inflammation and immune system dysregulation.

Symptoms:
- Nasal obstruction, sinus pain, and visible masses in the affected area.

Treatments:
- Medical: Radiation therapy is the primary treatment, with chemotherapy reserved for cases associated with multiple myeloma.
- Natural/Supportive: Anti-inflammatory diets and breathing exercises for symptom management.

Prevention:
- No established prevention, though regular monitoring for high-risk individuals (e.g., those with multiple myeloma) is recommended.

Global Perspective:
- Rare globally, with most cases reported in older adults. Access to radiation therapy is critical for treatment.

Personal Story:
Victor, a 63-year-old retired musician, underwent radiation therapy for extramedullary plasmacytoma. His recovery inspired him to create music promoting cancer awareness.


Part IV: The Cancers A-Z Directory

Continued: F

## 1. Fallopian Tube Cancer

**Definition:**
Fallopian tube cancer is a rare gynecologic cancer that begins in the fallopian tubes, the structures connecting the ovaries to the uterus. It is often linked to high-grade serous ovarian cancer due to overlapping characteristics.

**History:**
- First recognized as a distinct cancer in the 19th century.
- Advances in genetic testing (e.g., BRCA1/2 mutations) have improved early detection and prevention strategies.

**Causes:**
- Mutations in BRCA1 or BRCA2 genes.
- Risk factors include a family history of ovarian or breast cancer and conditions like pelvic inflammatory disease.

**Symptoms:**
- Abdominal or pelvic pain, abnormal vaginal bleeding, and bloating.

Treatments:
- Medical: Surgery (salpingo-oophorectomy), chemotherapy, and targeted therapies like PARP inhibitors.
- Natural/Supportive: Anti-inflammatory diets and yoga to reduce treatment-related fatigue.

Prevention:
- Risk-reducing salpingo-oophorectomy for BRCA mutation carriers.
- Regular gynecological exams and genetic counseling.

Global Perspective:
- Rare worldwide, with better outcomes in countries offering genetic testing and early intervention.
- Limited awareness in low-income regions often leads to delayed diagnoses.

Personal Story:
Karen, a 42-year-old genetic counselor, underwent preventive surgery after discovering she carried a BRCA1 mutation. Her advocacy for genetic testing has helped countless women make informed health decisions.

## 2. Fibrosarcoma

**Definition:**
Fibrosarcoma is a rare cancer that develops in fibroblasts, the connective tissue cells. It typically occurs in the limbs, trunk, or retroperitoneum.

**History:**
- First identified as a distinct cancer in the late 19th century.
- Advances in surgical techniques and targeted therapies have improved outcomes.

**Causes:**
- Genetic mutations in fibroblast cells.
- Risk factors include previous radiation therapy and hereditary conditions like Li-Fraumeni syndrome.

**Symptoms:**
- A painless lump or swelling in the affected area.
- Pain and restricted movement as the tumor grows.

**Treatments:**

- **Medical:** Surgery with wide margins, radiation therapy, and chemotherapy for advanced cases.
- **Natural/Supportive:** Physical therapy to regain mobility and dietary support to enhance recovery.

Prevention:
- Regular monitoring for individuals with genetic predispositions.

Global Perspective:
- Treated primarily in specialized cancer centers in high-income countries.
- Delayed diagnosis is common in low-income regions, leading to advanced-stage presentations.

Personal Story:
Mark, a 37-year-old carpenter, underwent limb-sparing surgery for fibrosarcoma in his thigh. His recovery journey inspired him to volunteer for cancer awareness programs in his community.

## 3. Follicular Lymphoma

Definition:

Follicular lymphoma is a slow-growing type of non-Hodgkin lymphoma that originates in B-cells. It often affects older adults and is considered indolent, though it can transform into more aggressive forms.

History:
- First described in the 20th century.
- Advances in immunotherapy and targeted treatments have improved outcomes.

Causes:
- Genetic mutations in B-cells, often involving the BCL2 gene.
- Risk factors include age, immunosuppression, and family history.

Symptoms:
- Enlarged lymph nodes, fatigue, night sweats, and unexplained weight loss.

Treatments:
- Medical: Rituximab (monoclonal antibody), chemotherapy, and radiation therapy.
- Natural/Supportive: Stress reduction techniques and balanced diets to maintain strength during treatment.

Prevention:
- No definitive prevention, though regular health check-ups can aid early detection.

Global Perspective:
- More prevalent in Western countries, with advanced therapies improving survival rates.
- Limited access to rituximab in low-income regions reduces treatment success.

Personal Story:
Eleanor, a 63-year-old grandmother, has managed her follicular lymphoma for over a decade with a combination of targeted therapy and lifestyle changes. She shares her journey through public speaking engagements.

4. Fetal Adenocarcinoma (Pulmonary)

Definition:
Fetal adenocarcinoma is a rare subtype of lung cancer characterized by gland-like structures resembling fetal lung tissue. It is a

variant of adenocarcinoma and primarily affects younger patients.

History:
- Recognized as a distinct subtype in the 20th century.
- Research into its unique genetic mutations continues to evolve.

Causes:
- Genetic mutations in EGFR or other oncogenes.
- No clear environmental or lifestyle risk factors, though smoking may contribute in some cases.

Symptoms:
- Persistent cough, shortness of breath, and chest pain.

Treatments:
- Medical: Surgery for localized tumors, targeted therapies, and chemotherapy.
- Natural/Supportive: Breathing exercises and dietary adjustments to improve lung health.

Prevention:

- Avoidance of smoking and secondhand smoke exposure.

Global Perspective:
- Rare globally, with better outcomes in regions with advanced diagnostic tools.

Personal Story:
Lila, a 28-year-old non-smoker, was diagnosed with fetal adenocarcinoma after persistent respiratory symptoms. Her successful treatment with targeted therapy inspired her to advocate for lung cancer awareness in younger populations.

## 5. Fibrolamellar Hepatocellular Carcinoma (FLHCC)

Definition:
Fibrolamellar hepatocellular carcinoma is a rare liver cancer that typically affects young adults without underlying liver disease.

History:
- First identified as a distinct subtype of liver cancer in the 20th century.
- Advances in surgical techniques have improved outcomes for localized cases.

Causes:
- Genetic mutations, particularly involving DNAJB1-PRKACA fusion.
- Unlike most liver cancers, it is not linked to alcohol use or viral hepatitis.

Symptoms:
- Abdominal pain, a palpable mass, and jaundice in advanced cases.

Treatments:
- Medical: Surgical resection is the primary treatment, with chemotherapy or targeted therapies for advanced cases.
- Natural/Supportive: Dietary support to improve liver function and reduce inflammation.

Prevention:
- No known prevention methods due to its genetic origin.

Global Perspective:
- Rare worldwide, with outcomes dependent on access to specialized surgical care.

Personal Story:

Jared, a 21-year-old athlete, underwent surgery for FLHCC after experiencing unexplained abdominal pain. His story inspired his local community to raise funds for liver cancer research.

## Part IV: The Cancers A-Z Directory

### Continued: G

### 1. Gallbladder Cancer

**Definition:**
Gallbladder cancer is a rare cancer that begins in the gallbladder, a small organ under the liver that stores bile. It is often diagnosed at advanced stages due to a lack of early symptoms.

**History:**
- Documented as early as the 18th century.
- Advances in imaging, such as ultrasound and CT scans, have improved diagnosis.

**Causes:**

- Chronic gallbladder inflammation due to gallstones or infections.
- Risk factors include obesity, a high-fat diet, and exposure to certain industrial chemicals.

Symptoms:
- Abdominal pain, jaundice, nausea, and unexplained weight loss.

Treatments:
- Medical: Surgery (cholecystectomy), chemotherapy, and radiation for advanced cases.
- Natural/Supportive: Liver-supporting diets and turmeric for its potential anti-inflammatory properties.

Prevention:
- Managing risk factors such as gallstones through a healthy diet and regular check-ups.

Global Perspective:
- High prevalence in regions like Chile, Bolivia, and India, linked to dietary and genetic factors.

- Limited treatment access in low-income areas contributes to poor survival rates.

Personal Story:
Rita, a 62-year-old woman from India, was diagnosed with gallbladder cancer after experiencing persistent abdominal pain. Her story highlights the importance of early detection in high-risk regions.

## 2. Gastric (Stomach) Cancer

Definition:
Gastric cancer develops in the lining of the stomach. It is often associated with Helicobacter pylori infection, dietary factors, and genetic predisposition.

History:
- Documented since ancient times, with significant advancements in treatment occurring in the 20th century.
- The link between H. pylori infection and gastric cancer was established in the 1980s.

Causes:

- H. pylori infection, diets high in smoked or salted foods, tobacco use, and chronic gastritis.
- Genetic mutations and syndromes such as Lynch syndrome also increase risk.

Symptoms:
- Indigestion, nausea, weight loss, and abdominal discomfort. Advanced stages may cause vomiting and difficulty swallowing.

Treatments:
- Medical: Surgery (gastrectomy), chemotherapy, radiation, and targeted therapies like trastuzumab for HER2-positive cases.
- Natural/Supportive: Probiotics for gut health and anti-inflammatory diets.

Prevention:
- H. pylori eradication through antibiotics.
- Diets rich in fresh fruits, vegetables, and fiber.

Global Perspective:
- High incidence in East Asia, particularly Japan and Korea, due to dietary factors and H. pylori prevalence.

- Screening programs in these countries have significantly improved early detection and survival rates.

Personal Story:
Kenji, a 58-year-old chef from Japan, was diagnosed with early-stage gastric cancer during a routine endoscopy. After a successful surgery, he became an advocate for regular screenings.

## 3. Gastrointestinal Stromal Tumor (GIST)

Definition:
GIST is a rare type of tumor that originates in the digestive tract's connective tissue, most commonly in the stomach or small intestine.

History:
- First identified as a distinct tumor type in the late 20th century.
- Advances in molecular biology led to the development of targeted therapies like imatinib.

Causes:
- Genetic mutations in the KIT or PDGFRA genes.

- No clear environmental or lifestyle risk factors.

Symptoms:
- Abdominal pain, gastrointestinal bleeding, and anemia.

Treatments:
- Medical: Surgery for localized tumors, with imatinib as a targeted therapy for advanced or metastatic cases.
- Natural/Supportive: Anti-inflammatory diets and stress management to support overall health.

Prevention:
- No known prevention methods due to its genetic origin.

Global Perspective:
- Rare worldwide, with outcomes dependent on access to targeted therapies.
- In low-income regions, the high cost of drugs like imatinib limits availability.

Personal Story:
Amara, a 42-year-old teacher from Kenya, struggled to access treatment for her GIST.

With the help of a global charity, she received targeted therapy and now raises awareness about rare cancers in underserved communities.

## 4. Germ Cell Tumors

Definition:
Germ cell tumors develop from reproductive cells and can occur in the testes, ovaries, or extragonadal locations like the chest or abdomen.

History:
- Germ cell tumors have been studied extensively since the 20th century, with significant advances in chemotherapy improving survival rates.

Causes:
- Genetic mutations in germ cells.
- Risk factors include undescended testicles and genetic syndromes like Klinefelter syndrome.

Symptoms:
- Swelling or pain in the affected area, fatigue, and unexplained weight loss.

Treatments:
- Medical: Surgery, chemotherapy (e.g., cisplatin-based regimens), and radiation therapy.
- Natural/Supportive: Balanced diets to support recovery and mindfulness techniques for emotional well-being.

Prevention:
- Regular self-exams for testicular tumors and prompt medical attention for abnormalities.

Global Perspective:
- Higher incidence of testicular germ cell tumors in Western countries.
- Access to advanced treatments has led to high survival rates in developed regions.

Personal Story:
Liam, a 22-year-old athlete from Canada, successfully overcame a testicular germ cell tumor. His journey inspired a campaign encouraging young men to prioritize their health.

5. Glioblastoma Multiforme (GBM)

Definition:

GBM is the most aggressive and common primary brain cancer, arising from glial cells. It grows rapidly and is challenging to treat.

History:
- First identified in the 20th century, with significant advancements in surgical techniques and radiation therapy in recent decades.

Causes:
- Genetic mutations in glial cells.
- Risk factors include previous radiation exposure and genetic syndromes like Li-Fraumeni.

Symptoms:
- Persistent headaches, seizures, cognitive impairments, and personality changes.

Treatments:
- Medical: Surgery, radiation, and chemotherapy with temozolomide. Emerging treatments include tumor-treating fields and immunotherapy.
- Natural/Supportive: Diets emphasizing brain health (e.g., omega-3 fatty acids) and physical therapy for rehabilitation.

Prevention:
- Limited prevention options due to its sporadic nature.

Global Perspective:
- Survival rates are low globally, but access to advanced care improves outcomes in developed nations.

Personal Story:
Laura, a 45-year-old writer, was diagnosed with GBM. Her experience inspired her to pen a memoir that raised awareness about the emotional challenges of living with brain cancer.

## Part IV: The Cancers A-Z Directory

Continued: H

1. Hairy Cell Leukemia (HCL)

Definition:
Hairy cell leukemia (HCL) is a rare, slow-growing cancer of the blood and bone marrow, named for the "hairy" appearance of

the abnormal B-lymphocytes under a microscope.

History:
- First identified in the mid-20th century.
- Advances in targeted therapies, such as cladribine, have greatly improved survival rates.

Causes:
- Genetic mutations in B-cells, specifically in the BRAF gene in most cases.
- No known environmental or hereditary risk factors.

Symptoms:
- Fatigue, frequent infections, easy bruising, and an enlarged spleen.

Treatments:
- Medical: Chemotherapy (cladribine or pentostatin), monoclonal antibodies (e.g., rituximab), and targeted therapies for BRAF mutations.
- Natural/Supportive: Balanced diets and moderate exercise to enhance immunity.

Prevention:

- No known prevention due to its genetic origin.

Global Perspective:
- More common in men than women, typically affecting older adults.
- Access to targeted therapies has significantly improved outcomes in developed countries.

Personal Story:
Peter, a 60-year-old accountant, was diagnosed with HCL after experiencing persistent fatigue. He credits targeted therapy with allowing him to continue his active lifestyle and pursue advocacy work.

2. Head and Neck Cancers

Definition:
Head and neck cancers encompass a group of cancers that originate in the mouth, throat, larynx, nasal cavity, or salivary glands. Most are squamous cell carcinomas.

History:
- Documented in ancient medical texts, with modern surgical and radiation techniques improving treatment outcomes.

- The link between HPV infection and throat cancer was established in the late 20th century.

Causes:
- Tobacco and alcohol use are the leading causes.
- Human papillomavirus (HPV) infection is a significant risk factor for oropharyngeal cancers.

Symptoms:
- A persistent sore throat, difficulty swallowing, hoarseness, and lumps in the neck.

Treatments:
- Medical: Surgery, radiation therapy, chemotherapy, and immunotherapy (e.g., pembrolizumab for advanced cases).
- Natural/Supportive: Speech therapy, anti-inflammatory diets, and herbal teas to soothe throat irritation.

Prevention:
- Avoiding tobacco and excessive alcohol consumption.

- HPV vaccination and regular oral health check-ups.

Global Perspective:
- Higher incidence in regions with high tobacco and alcohol consumption, such as South Asia.
- Public health campaigns have successfully reduced rates in some Western countries through HPV vaccination.

Personal Story:
Maria, a 45-year-old singer, underwent surgery and radiation for vocal cord cancer. Her recovery journey inspired her to create a support group for artists facing head and neck cancers.

## 3. Hepatocellular Carcinoma (HCC)

Definition:
Hepatocellular carcinoma (HCC) is the most common type of primary liver cancer, often linked to chronic liver disease and cirrhosis.

History:

- Documented in ancient Chinese and Greek texts, with modern understanding advanced by the discovery of viral hepatitis.
- The introduction of antiviral therapies has reduced the risk of HCC in high-risk populations.

Causes:
- Chronic infection with Hepatitis B or C viruses, excessive alcohol consumption, and non-alcoholic fatty liver disease (NAFLD).
- Exposure to aflatoxins, common in contaminated grains and nuts in certain regions.

Symptoms:
- Abdominal pain, jaundice, weight loss, and a palpable mass in the liver area.

Treatments:
- Medical: Surgery, liver transplantation, ablation, chemotherapy, targeted therapies (e.g., sorafenib), and immunotherapy.
- Natural/Supportive: Liver-friendly diets and lifestyle changes to reduce disease progression.

Prevention:

- Vaccination against Hepatitis B and antiviral treatments for Hepatitis C.
- Limiting alcohol intake and addressing obesity-related liver disease.

Global Perspective:
- High prevalence in Asia and Africa due to Hepatitis B and aflatoxin exposure.
- Screening programs in high-risk regions have improved early detection.

Personal Story:
Li Wei, a 50-year-old farmer from China, received a liver transplant for advanced HCC. His recovery inspired him to advocate for vaccination campaigns in rural areas.

## 4. Hodgkin Lymphoma (HL)

Definition:
Hodgkin lymphoma (HL) is a cancer of the lymphatic system characterized by the presence of Reed-Sternberg cells. It typically affects young adults and individuals over 55.

History:
- First described by Thomas Hodgkin in 1832.

- Advances in chemotherapy and radiation therapy in the 20th century drastically improved survival rates.

Causes:
- Exact cause unknown, but risk factors include Epstein-Barr virus (EBV) infection and a family history of lymphoma.

Symptoms:
- Painless swelling of lymph nodes, fever, night sweats, and unexplained weight loss.

Treatments:
- Medical: Chemotherapy (ABVD regimen), radiation therapy, and immunotherapy (e.g., brentuximab vedotin).
- Natural/Supportive: Stress management and nutrition to maintain energy during treatment.

Prevention:
- No established prevention, though managing EBV infections may reduce risk.

Global Perspective:
- High cure rates in developed countries due to effective therapies.

- Limited access to advanced treatments in low-income regions results in poorer outcomes.

Personal Story:
Jacob, your brother, successfully battled Hodgkin lymphoma and now inspires others with his story of resilience and hope.

5. Hypopharyngeal Cancer

Definition:
Hypopharyngeal cancer develops in the hypopharynx, the part of the throat near the larynx. It is a rare but aggressive form of head and neck cancer.

History:
- Advances in surgical and radiation techniques in the 20th century improved survival rates.

Causes:
- Tobacco and alcohol use are the primary risk factors.
- Nutritional deficiencies and HPV infection may also play a role.

Symptoms:
- Persistent sore throat, difficulty swallowing, and a lump in the neck.

Treatments:
- Medical: Surgery, radiation, and chemotherapy. Emerging treatments include immunotherapy for advanced cases.
- Natural/Supportive: Voice therapy and nutrient-dense diets to support healing.

Prevention:
- Avoiding tobacco and alcohol, maintaining a healthy diet, and seeking early medical attention for persistent throat symptoms.

Global Perspective:
- More common in regions with high tobacco and alcohol consumption.
- Awareness campaigns in developed nations have reduced incidence rates.

Personal Story:
Carlos, a 52-year-old truck driver, successfully underwent surgery for hypopharyngeal cancer and now advocates

for tobacco cessation programs in his community.

## Part IV: The Cancers A-Z Directory

Continued: I

### 1. Inflammatory Breast Cancer (IBC)

Definition:
Inflammatory breast cancer (IBC) is a rare and aggressive form of breast cancer that blocks lymph vessels in the skin of the breast, causing swelling and redness rather than a distinct lump.

History:
- First identified in the 19th century, IBC remains one of the most aggressive breast cancer types.
- Advances in multimodal treatments (combining chemotherapy, surgery, and radiation) have improved outcomes.

Causes:
- Genetic mutations in breast cells.

- Risk factors include obesity, hormone replacement therapy, and a family history of breast cancer.

Symptoms:
- Red, swollen, and warm breast with thickened skin resembling an orange peel.
- Rapid progression over weeks or months.

Treatments:
- Medical: Neoadjuvant chemotherapy (before surgery), mastectomy, radiation therapy, and targeted therapies like trastuzumab for HER2-positive cases.
- Natural/Supportive: Nutritional support to maintain energy during treatment and lymphatic massage to manage swelling.

Prevention:
- Maintaining a healthy weight and minimizing hormone replacement therapy risks.
- Early recognition of symptoms for prompt treatment.

Global Perspective:
- More common in younger women and African American populations.

- Survival rates are improving with access to comprehensive cancer centers in developed nations.

Personal Story:
Tasha, a 38-year-old mother of two, overcame IBC with aggressive treatment and now leads a support group for young women facing breast cancer.

## 2. Intrahepatic Cholangiocarcinoma

Definition:
Intrahepatic cholangiocarcinoma is a type of bile duct cancer that originates within the liver. It is rare but often diagnosed at advanced stages.

History:
- Advances in imaging and molecular profiling in the late 20th century have improved early detection and treatment options.

Causes:
- Chronic liver conditions like hepatitis B or C, cirrhosis, or liver fluke infections.
- Genetic mutations and exposure to certain chemicals (e.g., nitrosamines).

Symptoms:
- Jaundice, abdominal pain, unexplained weight loss, and dark urine.

Treatments:
- Medical: Surgery (liver resection), chemotherapy, targeted therapies (e.g., FGFR inhibitors), and liver transplantation.
- Natural/Supportive: Diets low in fat and alcohol avoidance to support liver health.

Prevention:
- Vaccination against hepatitis B and management of chronic liver diseases.
- Proper cooking of freshwater fish in regions with endemic liver fluke infections.

Global Perspective:
- High prevalence in Southeast Asia due to liver fluke infections.
- Advanced treatments in developed nations have improved survival rates.

Personal Story:
Vila, a 50-year-old from Thailand, underwent surgery for cholangiocarcinoma after a diagnosis linked to liver fluke exposure. Her story highlights the importance of public health interventions in high-risk areas.

## 3. Intestinal Cancer

Definition:
Intestinal cancer develops in the small intestine, a rare form of gastrointestinal cancer compared to colon or stomach cancer.

History:
- Historically overshadowed by other gastrointestinal cancers, but recent advancements in endoscopy have improved diagnosis.

Causes:
- Genetic mutations (e.g., APC gene in familial adenomatous polyposis).
- Risk factors include Crohn's disease, celiac disease, and diets high in red meat and processed foods.

Symptoms:
- Abdominal pain, nausea, weight loss, and gastrointestinal bleeding.

Treatments:

- **Medical:** Surgery (resection of the affected intestine), chemotherapy, and targeted therapies for advanced cases.
- **Natural/Supportive:** Anti-inflammatory diets and probiotics to support gut health.

**Prevention:**
- Managing chronic gastrointestinal conditions and adopting a high-fiber diet.

**Global Perspective:**
- Rare globally, with better outcomes in regions with advanced diagnostic tools.

**Personal Story:**
Clara, a 45-year-old nutritionist, was diagnosed with intestinal cancer after years of Crohn's disease. Her treatment journey inspired her to educate others about managing chronic GI conditions.

## 4. Intraductal Papillary Mucinous Neoplasm (IPMN)

**Definition:**
IPMN is a type of pancreatic cystic tumor that can progress to pancreatic cancer if untreated.

History:
- First described in the late 20th century as a precursor to invasive pancreatic cancer.

Causes:
- Genetic mutations in pancreatic cells.
- Risk factors include chronic pancreatitis, diabetes, and family history of pancreatic cancer.

Symptoms:
- Abdominal pain, weight loss, and jaundice in advanced cases. Often asymptomatic in early stages.

Treatments:
- Medical: Surgery (pancreaticoduodenectomy) for high-risk lesions, with surveillance for low-risk cases.
- Natural/Supportive: Low-fat diets to reduce pancreatic strain.

Prevention:
- Regular screenings for individuals with a family history or hereditary syndromes.

- Lifestyle changes to reduce diabetes and pancreatitis risk.

Global Perspective:
- More common in older adults. Access to specialized surgical centers is critical for optimal outcomes.

Personal Story:
Martin, a 60-year-old retiree, underwent surgery for IPMN after an incidental finding during a health check-up. His experience emphasized the value of regular screenings for early detection.

## 5. Iris Melanoma

Definition:
Iris melanoma is a rare eye cancer that develops in the pigmented cells of the iris. It is usually slow-growing but can spread to other parts of the body.

History:
- Identified as a distinct type of uveal melanoma in the 20th century.
- Advances in ocular oncology have improved diagnosis and treatment.

Causes:

- Mutations in genes like GNAQ and GNA11.
- Risk factors include fair skin, light-colored eyes, and excessive UV exposure.

Symptoms:
- A dark spot on the iris, vision changes, or eye pain.

Treatments:
- Medical: Observation for small tumors, radiation therapy, or surgery for larger tumors. Enucleation (removal of the eye) may be required in advanced cases.
- Natural/Supportive: Protective eyewear to reduce UV exposure and antioxidants for eye health.

Prevention:
- Regular eye exams, especially for individuals with light-colored eyes.
- Avoiding excessive sun exposure.

Global Perspective:
- Rare worldwide, with higher incidence in fair-skinned populations.

Personal Story:
Ella, a 32-year-old artist, noticed a dark spot on her iris during a routine eye exam. Early

treatment preserved her vision, and she now creates artwork inspired by her journey.

## Part IV: The Cancers A-Z Directory

### Continued: J

#### 1. Jaw Cancer (Oral and Maxillofacial Cancer)

**Definition:**
Jaw cancer refers to malignancies that develop in the jawbone or surrounding tissues. It is often associated with oral cancers affecting the gums, tongue, or floor of the mouth.

**History:**
- Documented in ancient medical texts, with significant advancements in surgical and reconstructive techniques occurring in the 20th century.

**Causes:**
- Tobacco use, heavy alcohol consumption, poor oral hygiene, and human papillomavirus (HPV) infection.
- Prolonged exposure to carcinogens, such as betel quid chewing in South Asia, is a significant risk factor.

Symptoms:
- Persistent jaw pain, swelling, loose teeth, and difficulty chewing.
- In advanced stages, facial deformity or numbness may occur.

Treatments:
- Medical: Surgery to remove the tumor, often followed by radiation therapy and chemotherapy. Reconstructive surgery is often required.
- Natural/Supportive: Nutritional support through soft or liquid diets during recovery, and physical therapy for jaw mobility.

Prevention:
- Avoiding tobacco and alcohol, maintaining good oral hygiene, and receiving the HPV vaccine.

Global Perspective:
- Higher prevalence in South Asia and parts of Africa due to betel quid chewing and poor dental care access.
- Public health campaigns in these regions focus on tobacco cessation and oral cancer screenings.

**Personal Story:**
Rahul, a 46-year-old teacher from India, overcame jaw cancer after undergoing surgery and radiation. He now educates his community on the dangers of betel nut chewing and the importance of early detection.

## 2. Juvenile Myelomonocytic Leukemia (JMML)

**Definition:**
Juvenile myelomonocytic leukemia (JMML) is a rare and aggressive blood cancer that primarily affects children under the age of 4. It originates in the bone marrow and leads to the overproduction of immature white blood cells.

**History:**
- First described in the mid-20th century as a distinct pediatric leukemia subtype.
- Advances in genetic research have identified mutations like PTPN11 and NRAS as key drivers.

**Causes:**
- Genetic mutations in blood-forming cells.

- Often associated with hereditary conditions like Noonan syndrome or neurofibromatosis type 1 (NF1).

Symptoms:
- Pale skin, fever, frequent infections, enlarged spleen, and skin rashes.

Treatments:
- Medical: Hematopoietic stem cell transplantation (bone marrow transplant) is the only curative option. Supportive care includes blood transfusions and antibiotics.
- Natural/Supportive: Nutritional support to strengthen immunity and manage treatment side effects.

Prevention:
- No known prevention, though genetic counseling may help families with hereditary conditions.

Global Perspective:
- Rare worldwide, with better outcomes in regions offering access to stem cell transplantation.

Personal Story:
Liam, a 3-year-old from the UK, underwent a successful stem cell transplant for JMML. His

parents now advocate for increased awareness of rare pediatric cancers and the importance of donor registries.

## 3. Juvenile Pilocytic Astrocytoma (JPA)

Definition:
Juvenile pilocytic astrocytoma is a slow-growing brain tumor primarily affecting children and young adults. It often arises in the cerebellum or optic pathways.

History:
- First identified in the 20th century, JPAs are now recognized as one of the most common pediatric brain tumors.
- Advances in MRI technology have improved early detection and surgical precision.

Causes:
- Genetic mutations in the MAPK pathway, often involving the BRAF gene.
- No clear environmental or hereditary risk factors.

Symptoms:
- Headaches, balance issues, nausea, and vision changes.

Treatments:
- Medical: Surgery is often curative for localized tumors. Chemotherapy and targeted therapies are options for inoperable cases.
- Natural/Supportive: Occupational therapy and cognitive rehabilitation to address neurological deficits.

Prevention:
- No known prevention due to its genetic nature.

Global Perspective:
- High survival rates in developed nations due to advanced surgical techniques.
- In resource-limited regions, delayed diagnosis often leads to complications.

Personal Story:
Sophia, a 10-year-old gymnast, underwent surgery for a JPA in her cerebellum. Her successful recovery allowed her to return to gymnastics, inspiring her peers with her resilience.

4. Juvenile Polyposis Syndrome (JPS)-Associated Cancer

**Definition:**
Juvenile polyposis syndrome (JPS) is a hereditary condition that causes multiple polyps in the gastrointestinal tract, increasing the risk of colorectal and stomach cancer.

**History:**
- First described in the early 20th century, with the genetic basis (SMAD4 or BMPR1A mutations) identified in recent decades.

**Causes:**
- Mutations in the SMAD4 or BMPR1A genes.
- Familial inheritance in most cases.

**Symptoms:**
- Gastrointestinal bleeding, anemia, and abdominal pain.

**Treatments:**
- Medical: Regular polyp removal via endoscopy and surgery for advanced cases. Surveillance programs are critical for early cancer detection.

- **Natural/Supportive:** High-fiber diets and probiotics to support gastrointestinal health.

Prevention:
- Genetic counseling and regular screenings for at-risk individuals.

Global Perspective:
- Rare worldwide, with outcomes highly dependent on access to genetic testing and surveillance.

Personal Story:
Emma, a 15-year-old diagnosed with JPS, undergoes regular screenings and polyp removal. Her family's proactive approach has inspired others to prioritize genetic counseling and early intervention.

## Part IV: The Cancers A-Z Directory

Continued: K

1. Kaposi Sarcoma (KS)

Definition:

Kaposi sarcoma is a cancer that forms in the lining of blood and lymphatic vessels. It often appears as purple, red, or brown lesions on the skin, but it can also affect internal organs. It is strongly associated with human herpesvirus 8 (HHV-8) infection.

History:
- First described by dermatologist Moritz Kaposi in 1872.
- Became widely recognized during the HIV/AIDS epidemic in the 1980s as an AIDS-related cancer.

Causes:
- HHV-8 infection is a necessary cause.
- Immunosuppression, as seen in HIV/AIDS or organ transplant patients, increases risk.

Symptoms:
- Skin lesions that may bleed or ulcerate.
- Swelling in the legs and difficulty breathing if internal organs are involved.

Treatments:

- Medical: Antiretroviral therapy (ART) for HIV-associated KS, chemotherapy, and radiation therapy.
- Natural/Supportive: Nutritional support to strengthen immunity and reduce inflammation.

Prevention:
- Managing HIV/AIDS with ART.
- Avoiding HHV-8 transmission through safe sexual practices and blood screening.

Global Perspective:
- More common in sub-Saharan Africa, where HHV-8 and HIV rates are high.
- ART has dramatically reduced KS cases in developed nations.

Personal Story:
Michael, a 35-year-old from Kenya, received ART and chemotherapy for KS. His recovery inspired him to become an HIV/AIDS educator in his community.

2. Kidney Cancer (Renal Cell Carcinoma)

Definition:

Kidney cancer, most commonly renal cell carcinoma (RCC), originates in the small tubules of the kidney. Other types include transitional cell carcinoma and Wilms tumor (in children).

History:
- First classified as a distinct cancer type in the 19th century.
- Advances in imaging and targeted therapies have improved outcomes.

Causes:
- Smoking, obesity, hypertension, and genetic syndromes like von Hippel-Lindau disease.
- Occupational exposure to chemicals such as cadmium.

Symptoms:
- Blood in the urine (hematuria), persistent back or flank pain, and unexplained weight loss.

Treatments:
- Medical: Surgery (nephrectomy), targeted therapies (e.g., sunitinib), immunotherapy (e.g., nivolumab), and ablation for smaller tumors.

- **Natural/Supportive:** Low-sodium diets and physical activity to support kidney health.

Prevention:
- Avoiding smoking, maintaining a healthy weight, and managing blood pressure.

Global Perspective:
- Higher incidence in developed nations, likely due to lifestyle factors and better diagnostic tools.
- Limited access to targeted therapies in low-income countries affects survival rates.

Personal Story:
Anna, a 55-year-old marathon runner, overcame kidney cancer with early surgery. She now advocates for regular health check-ups and cancer awareness.

## 3. Krukenberg Tumor

Definition:

A Krukenberg tumor is a rare metastatic ovarian tumor, usually originating from a primary cancer in the stomach, colon, or breast.

History:
- First described in 1896 by Friedrich Krukenberg.
- Understanding its metastatic nature has improved diagnostic accuracy.

Causes:
- Spread of primary cancers, particularly gastric cancer, through the lymphatic or blood systems.

Symptoms:
- Abdominal pain, bloating, and ascites (fluid buildup in the abdomen).

Treatments:
- Medical: Surgery to remove the ovaries and primary tumor, chemotherapy for systemic control.
- Natural/Supportive: Nutritional support to manage weight loss and fatigue.

Prevention:
- Early detection and treatment of primary cancers.

**Global Perspective:**
- More common in regions with high gastric cancer rates, such as East Asia.
- Delayed diagnosis is common due to the aggressive nature of metastasis.

**Personal Story:**
Mai, a 47-year-old from Japan, discovered a Krukenberg tumor during treatment for gastric cancer. Her story underscores the importance of comprehensive cancer care.

## 4. Keratoacanthoma

**Definition:**
Keratoacanthoma is a low-grade, rapidly growing skin tumor that resembles squamous cell carcinoma. It often resolves on its own but may require treatment to prevent recurrence.

**History:**
- First recognized as a distinct skin condition in the mid-20th century.
- Advances in dermatology have clarified its relationship with squamous cell carcinoma.

**Causes:**

- Prolonged sun exposure and weakened immune systems.
- Possible link to HPV infection.

Symptoms:
- A dome-shaped nodule with a central keratin-filled crater, typically on sun-exposed areas like the face or hands.

Treatments:
- Medical: Surgical excision, cryotherapy, or intralesional injections.
- Natural/Supportive: Sun protection and skincare to prevent further lesions.

Prevention:
- Consistent use of sunscreen and protective clothing.
- Regular skin checks for individuals with a history of skin tumors.

Global Perspective:
- More common in fair-skinned individuals and regions with high UV exposure.

Personal Story:
Sarah, a 62-year-old retiree, discovered keratoacanthoma on her nose. Prompt removal and regular skin checks helped her maintain her health and confidence.

# Part IV: The Cancers A-Z Directory

## Continued: L

### 1. Laryngeal Cancer

**Definition:**
Laryngeal cancer originates in the tissues of the larynx (voice box). It is most commonly squamous cell carcinoma.

**History:**
- First documented in the 19th century, with surgical interventions improving survival rates significantly over time.
- Modern treatments, such as larynx-preserving therapies, have advanced patient outcomes.

**Causes:**
- Smoking, heavy alcohol consumption, and human papillomavirus (HPV) infection.
- Exposure to occupational hazards like asbestos and wood dust.

**Symptoms:**

- Hoarseness, difficulty swallowing, persistent sore throat, and a lump in the neck.

Treatments:
- Medical: Surgery, radiation therapy, chemotherapy, and targeted therapy for advanced cases.
- Natural/Supportive: Speech therapy and anti-inflammatory diets to manage symptoms and recovery.

Prevention:
- Avoiding tobacco and excessive alcohol consumption.
- HPV vaccination and protective measures in hazardous workplaces.

Global Perspective:
- Higher prevalence in regions with high smoking and alcohol use, such as parts of Eastern Europe and South Asia.
- Early detection and treatment improve outcomes significantly.

Personal Story:

James, a 58-year-old actor, underwent surgery and voice therapy for laryngeal cancer. His recovery enabled him to continue his acting career, inspiring others in the arts.

## 2. Leukemia (General Overview)

**Definition:**
Leukemia is a cancer of the blood and bone marrow, characterized by the abnormal proliferation of white blood cells. It is classified into acute or chronic forms and lymphoid or myeloid types.

**History:**
- First described in the 19th century as a "white blood disease."
- Advances in chemotherapy and bone marrow transplants have transformed leukemia from a fatal disease to one with high survival rates for many patients.

**Causes:**
- Genetic mutations in blood-forming cells.
- Risk factors include exposure to radiation, certain chemicals, and genetic disorders like Down syndrome.

**Symptoms:**

- Fatigue, frequent infections, bruising, bleeding, and bone pain.

Treatments:
- Medical: Chemotherapy, targeted therapies, immunotherapy, and stem cell transplantation.
- Natural/Supportive: Diets rich in antioxidants, physical therapy, and stress-reducing practices.

Prevention:
- Avoiding known carcinogens and managing inherited risk factors.

Global Perspective:
- High survival rates for childhood leukemia in developed nations.
- Limited access to advanced treatments in low-income countries leads to poorer outcomes.

Personal Story:
Sophia, a 7-year-old leukemia survivor, underwent a successful bone marrow transplant and now inspires others with her journey of resilience and strength.

3. Liver Cancer

Definition:
Liver cancer typically refers to hepatocellular carcinoma (HCC), although other types include intrahepatic cholangiocarcinoma and angiosarcoma.

History:
- Descriptions of liver tumors date back to ancient Egypt.
- Vaccination against Hepatitis B and antiviral treatments for Hepatitis C have significantly reduced liver cancer rates in high-risk populations.

Causes:
- Chronic hepatitis B or C infection, heavy alcohol use, aflatoxin exposure, and non-alcoholic fatty liver disease (NAFLD).
- Cirrhosis, often caused by these factors, is a major risk for liver cancer.

Symptoms:
- Abdominal pain, jaundice, nausea, and unexplained weight loss.

Treatments:
- Medical: Surgery, liver transplantation, targeted therapies (e.g., sorafenib), and immunotherapy.

- **Natural/Supportive:** Diets low in fat and alcohol-free lifestyles to support liver health.

Prevention:
- Vaccination for hepatitis B, antiviral treatment for hepatitis C, and dietary measures to reduce aflatoxin exposure.

Global Perspective:
- High prevalence in sub-Saharan Africa and Asia due to hepatitis and aflatoxin exposure.
- Early detection and treatment improve outcomes in regions with access to advanced care.

Personal Story:
Ahmed, a 52-year-old farmer from Nigeria, received surgery for HCC after a diagnosis linked to aflatoxin exposure. His recovery inspired local awareness campaigns about food safety.

4. Lung Cancer

Definition:
Lung cancer is the leading cause of cancer-related deaths worldwide, primarily caused

by smoking and environmental exposures. The two main types are non-small cell lung cancer (NSCLC) and small cell lung cancer (SCLC).

History:
- Linked to smoking in the mid-20th century, with public health campaigns significantly reducing incidence in some regions.
- Advances in targeted therapies and immunotherapy have improved outcomes for advanced cases.

Causes:
- Smoking is the leading cause, along with radon exposure, air pollution, and occupational hazards like asbestos.
- Genetic mutations, particularly in EGFR, ALK, or KRAS, play a role in some cases.

Symptoms:
- Persistent cough, chest pain, shortness of breath, and unexplained weight loss.

Treatments:
- Medical: Surgery, radiation, chemotherapy, targeted therapies (e.g.,

osimertinib), and immunotherapy (e.g., pembrolizumab).
- Natural/Supportive: Breathing exercises, anti-inflammatory diets, and mindfulness practices.

Prevention:
- Avoiding tobacco and secondhand smoke, testing for radon, and using protective gear in hazardous workplaces.

Global Perspective:
- Smoking rates strongly correlate with lung cancer incidence, with higher rates in countries with lax tobacco regulations.
- Access to advanced treatments remains limited in low-income regions.

Personal Story:
Carlos, a 65-year-old former smoker, overcame lung cancer with a combination of surgery and immunotherapy. His story highlights the power of quitting smoking and early detection.


Part IV: The Cancers A-Z Directory

Continued: M

# 1. Male Breast Cancer

**Definition:**
Male breast cancer is a rare cancer that develops in the breast tissue of men. It often presents similarly to breast cancer in women but is typically diagnosed at a later stage.

**History:**
- First documented in medical literature in the 19th century.
- Advances in awareness and imaging have improved early detection in recent years.

**Causes:**
- Genetic mutations, particularly in BRCA1 and BRCA2.
- Risk factors include radiation exposure, high estrogen levels, obesity, and a family history of breast cancer.

**Symptoms:**
- A lump in the breast, nipple discharge, or changes in the skin around the breast.

**Treatments:**
- Medical: Surgery (mastectomy), chemotherapy, radiation therapy, and

hormonal therapy (e.g., tamoxifen for hormone-receptor-positive cancers).
- Natural/Supportive: Balanced diets, physical activity, and support groups to address stigma.

Prevention:
- Genetic testing for high-risk individuals and maintaining a healthy weight.

Global Perspective:
- Rare worldwide, with higher detection rates in regions with robust screening programs.
- Limited awareness in low-income countries contributes to delayed diagnosis.

Personal Story:
John, a 62-year-old mechanic, was diagnosed with breast cancer after noticing a lump. His treatment and advocacy have helped raise awareness of male breast cancer in his community.

## 2. Medulloblastoma

Definition:

Medulloblastoma is a fast-growing brain tumor that originates in the cerebellum. It is most common in children and can spread to other parts of the central nervous system.

History:
- First described in the 1920s, with advancements in radiation and chemotherapy significantly improving survival rates.

Causes:
- Genetic mutations in pathways like WNT, SHH, and TP53.
- No clear environmental risk factors, though hereditary syndromes like Li-Fraumeni increase risk.

Symptoms:
- Headaches, nausea, balance issues, and difficulty walking.

Treatments:
- Medical: Surgery, radiation therapy (for older children), and chemotherapy. Emerging treatments include targeted therapies based on tumor subtypes.
- Natural/Supportive: Physical and occupational therapy to aid recovery.

**Prevention:**
- No known prevention, but genetic counseling is advised for families with hereditary syndromes.

**Global Perspective:**
- High survival rates in developed nations due to advanced treatments and pediatric oncology expertise.
- In low-income regions, delayed diagnosis often leads to worse outcomes.

**Personal Story:**
Emma, a 6-year-old from Canada, underwent surgery and chemotherapy for medulloblastoma. Her resilience inspired her family to fundraise for pediatric brain cancer research.

## 3. Melanoma

**Definition:**
Melanoma is an aggressive skin cancer that develops in melanocytes, the cells that produce pigment. It can spread rapidly to other parts of the body if not detected early.

History:
- Documented as a distinct cancer type in the early 19th century.
- Advances in immunotherapy and targeted treatments have improved outcomes for advanced cases.

Causes:
- Excessive UV exposure from sunlight or tanning beds.
- Genetic predisposition, particularly in fair-skinned individuals with many moles.

Symptoms:
- A mole that changes in size, shape, or color.
- Lesions that itch, bleed, or do not heal.

Treatments:
- Medical: Surgical excision for localized melanoma, immunotherapy (e.g., pembrolizumab), and targeted therapies for advanced cases.
- Natural/Supportive: Sunscreen use, protective clothing, and regular skin checks to prevent recurrence.

Prevention:

- Avoiding excessive sun exposure and tanning beds.
- Regular dermatologist visits for high-risk individuals.

Global Perspective:
- High prevalence in Australia and New Zealand due to intense UV exposure.
- Public health campaigns in these regions emphasize sun protection and early detection.

Personal Story:
Claire, a 35-year-old lifeguard, was diagnosed with early-stage melanoma. Her story inspired her community to adopt better sun safety practices.

4. Mesothelioma

Definition:
Mesothelioma is a rare cancer that develops in the lining of the lungs (pleura), abdomen (peritoneum), or heart (pericardium). It is strongly linked to asbestos exposure.

History:
- First described in the early 20th century.

- Awareness of asbestos risks led to bans in many countries during the late 20th century.

Causes:
- Prolonged inhalation or ingestion of asbestos fibers.
- Risk increases with occupational exposure in industries like construction, shipbuilding, and mining.

Symptoms:
- Shortness of breath, chest pain, and fluid buildup in the lungs.
- Abdominal swelling and pain for peritoneal mesothelioma.

Treatments:
- Medical: Surgery, chemotherapy (e.g., pemetrexed and cisplatin), and radiation. Emerging treatments include immunotherapy.
- Natural/Supportive: Breathing exercises and anti-inflammatory diets to alleviate symptoms.

Prevention:
- Avoiding asbestos exposure and ensuring safe removal in older buildings.

Global Perspective:
- Still prevalent in countries where asbestos use has not been banned.
- Early detection is rare, leading to poorer outcomes in low-income regions.

Personal Story:
Henry, a 70-year-old retired shipbuilder, developed pleural mesothelioma decades after asbestos exposure. His advocacy for workplace safety has brought attention to this preventable cancer.

## 5. Multiple Myeloma

Definition:
Multiple myeloma is a cancer of plasma cells, a type of white blood cell responsible for producing antibodies. It often affects multiple bones in the body.

History:
- First described in the 19th century, with significant treatment advancements occurring in the late 20th century.

Causes:
- Genetic mutations in plasma cells.

- Risk factors include age, obesity, and exposure to radiation or certain chemicals.

Symptoms:
- Bone pain, fractures, fatigue, frequent infections, and kidney dysfunction.

Treatments:
- Medical: Chemotherapy, stem cell transplantation, and targeted therapies like bortezomib and lenalidomide.
- Natural/Supportive: Bone-strengthening exercises, balanced diets, and hydration to support kidney health.

Prevention:
- No known prevention, but early detection improves outcomes.

Global Perspective:
- Higher incidence in African Americans compared to other populations.
- Access to advanced therapies remains limited in low-income countries.

Personal Story:
Linda, a 62-year-old grandmother, credits early treatment and a supportive care team

for managing her multiple myeloma and maintaining her quality of life.

## Part IV: The Cancers A-Z Directory

### Continued: N

### 1. Nasopharyngeal Cancer

**Definition:**
Nasopharyngeal cancer is a rare type of head and neck cancer that starts in the nasopharynx, the upper part of the throat behind the nose. It is often linked to Epstein-Barr virus (EBV) infection.

**History:**
- First recognized in the late 19th century.
- Advances in radiation therapy and chemotherapy have improved outcomes for advanced cases.

**Causes:**
- Epstein-Barr virus (EBV) infection, genetic predisposition, and consumption of salted or preserved foods high in nitrosamines.

- Tobacco and alcohol use are minor contributing factors.

Symptoms:
- Nasal congestion, nosebleeds, hearing loss, and lumps in the neck.

Treatments:
- Medical: Radiation therapy is the primary treatment, often combined with chemotherapy for advanced cases.
- Natural/Supportive: Breathing exercises and dietary changes to support overall health.

Prevention:
- Reducing intake of preserved foods and addressing EBV infections early.
- Regular check-ups for individuals in high-risk regions.

Global Perspective:
- High prevalence in southern China and Southeast Asia, known as the "Cantonese cancer."
- Early detection programs in high-risk areas have improved survival rates.

Personal Story:

Chen, a 45-year-old chef from Guangdong, overcame nasopharyngeal cancer through a combination of radiation and chemotherapy. His advocacy focuses on promoting EBV awareness and cancer screenings.

## 2. Neuroblastoma

**Definition:**
Neuroblastoma is a cancer that develops in immature nerve cells, primarily affecting infants and young children. It most commonly starts in the adrenal glands but can also occur along the spine.

**History:**
- First identified in the 19th century.
- Research into genetic mutations like ALK has led to targeted therapies.

**Causes:**
- Genetic mutations in neuroblasts.
- Hereditary neuroblastoma accounts for a small percentage of cases, often linked to ALK or PHOX2B gene mutations.

**Symptoms:**
- Abdominal swelling, fatigue, fever, and bone pain in advanced stages.

Treatments:
- Medical: Surgery, chemotherapy, radiation therapy, and immunotherapy. High-risk cases may require stem cell transplants.
- Natural/Supportive: Nutritional support and physical therapy during recovery.

Prevention:
- No known prevention due to its genetic origin.

Global Perspective:
- More common in children under 5 years old. Survival rates vary significantly based on access to advanced treatments.

Personal Story:
Maya, a 3-year-old from the U.S., received cutting-edge immunotherapy after being diagnosed with high-risk neuroblastoma. Her story has inspired increased funding for pediatric cancer research.

## 3. Non-Hodgkin Lymphoma (NHL)

Definition:
Non-Hodgkin lymphoma encompasses a diverse group of blood cancers that affect

lymphocytes. It is categorized by the type of lymphocyte involved (B-cell or T-cell) and its growth rate (indolent or aggressive).

History:
- Identified as a distinct group of lymphomas in the mid-20th century.
- Advances in targeted therapies and immunotherapy have significantly improved survival rates.

Causes:
- Genetic mutations in lymphocytes, infections (e.g., EBV, HIV, or H. pylori), and immunosuppression.
- Risk factors include age, exposure to certain chemicals, and autoimmune diseases.

Symptoms:
- Enlarged lymph nodes, fever, night sweats, weight loss, and fatigue.

Treatments:
- Medical: Chemotherapy (e.g., CHOP regimen), immunotherapy (e.g., rituximab), radiation, and stem cell transplants for refractory cases.

- Natural/Supportive: Stress-reducing practices like yoga, balanced diets, and regular exercise.

Prevention:
- Managing infections and avoiding exposure to known carcinogens.

Global Perspective:
- Incidence is rising globally, particularly in high-income countries.
- Disparities in treatment access lead to worse outcomes in low-income regions.

Personal Story:
David, a 60-year-old from the UK, achieved remission after immunotherapy for B-cell NHL. His journey highlights the importance of early detection and advanced treatments.

## 4. Non-Small Cell Lung Cancer (NSCLC)

Definition:
NSCLC accounts for about 85% of all lung cancer cases and includes subtypes like adenocarcinoma, squamous cell carcinoma, and large cell carcinoma.

History:
- Public health campaigns in the 20th century reduced smoking rates, decreasing NSCLC incidence.
- Advances in targeted therapies and immunotherapy have transformed treatment for advanced cases.

Causes:
- Smoking is the leading cause, followed by radon exposure, air pollution, and occupational hazards like asbestos.
- Genetic mutations, such as EGFR, ALK, or KRAS, drive some cases.

Symptoms:
- Persistent cough, chest pain, shortness of breath, and fatigue.

Treatments:
- Medical: Surgery for localized tumors, radiation therapy, chemotherapy, targeted therapies (e.g., osimertinib), and immunotherapy (e.g., pembrolizumab).
- Natural/Supportive: Breathing exercises, anti-inflammatory diets, and complementary therapies for symptom relief.

Prevention:

- Avoiding smoking, testing for radon, and protecting workers from hazardous substances.

Global Perspective:
- High incidence in countries with high smoking rates, such as China and Russia.
- Disparities in treatment access remain a challenge in low-income regions.

Personal Story:
Lena, a 58-year-old former smoker, responded well to targeted therapy for EGFR-mutated NSCLC. Her advocacy promotes early detection and quitting smoking.

## 5. Nodular Melanoma

Definition:
Nodular melanoma is an aggressive form of skin cancer that grows rapidly and penetrates deeper layers of the skin. It accounts for about 15% of melanoma cases but causes a disproportionate number of deaths.

History:
- First distinguished from other melanoma subtypes in the 20th century.

- Public health campaigns emphasize early detection to reduce mortality.

Causes:
- Excessive UV exposure, particularly in fair-skinned individuals.
- Genetic mutations like BRAF or NRAS in melanocytes.

Symptoms:
- A firm, raised, dark-colored bump that may ulcerate or bleed.

Treatments:
- Medical: Surgical excision, immunotherapy, and targeted therapies for advanced cases.
- Natural/Supportive: Regular skin checks and protective clothing to prevent recurrence.

Prevention:
- Avoiding tanning beds and protecting skin from excessive sun exposure.
- Regular dermatologist visits for high-risk individuals.

Global Perspective:

- High prevalence in Australia and New Zealand due to intense UV exposure.
- Early detection programs in these regions have improved survival rates.

Personal Story:
Jack, a 42-year-old outdoor enthusiast, survived nodular melanoma after aggressive treatment. His story inspires others to prioritize skin protection and regular check-ups.

## Part IV: The Cancers A-Z Directory

Continued: O

### 1. Ocular Melanoma

Definition:
Ocular melanoma is a rare cancer that develops in the melanocytes of the eye. It is the most common primary eye cancer in adults and typically arises in the uvea (the middle layer of the eye).

History:
- First recognized as a distinct type of melanoma in the 19th century.

- Advances in radiation therapy and enucleation techniques have improved treatment outcomes.

Causes:
- Genetic mutations, often involving the GNAQ and GNA11 genes.
- Risk factors include light-colored eyes, excessive UV exposure, and a family history of melanoma.

Symptoms:
- Blurry vision, a dark spot on the iris, or flashing lights in the visual field.
- Often asymptomatic in early stages, discovered during routine eye exams.

Treatments:
- Medical: Radiation therapy (e.g., plaque brachytherapy), surgery (enucleation for advanced cases), and targeted therapies in clinical trials.
- Natural/Supportive: Protective eyewear to reduce UV exposure and antioxidant-rich diets to support eye health.

Prevention:
- Regular eye exams, especially for individuals with light-colored eyes or a family history of melanoma.

- Reducing UV exposure with sunglasses and hats.

Global Perspective:
- Rare worldwide, with higher incidence in fair-skinned populations.
- Access to specialized ocular oncology centers is critical for effective treatment.

Personal Story:
Sophia, a 50-year-old artist, was diagnosed with ocular melanoma after noticing vision changes. Her treatment allowed her to continue her creative work and advocate for regular eye exams.

## 2. Oligodendroglioma

Definition:
Oligodendroglioma is a rare, slow-growing brain tumor that arises from oligodendrocytes, cells that produce the protective myelin sheath around nerves in the brain and spinal cord.

History:
- First described in the early 20th century.

- Advances in molecular profiling, particularly the identification of 1p/19q co-deletion, have improved diagnosis and treatment.

Causes:
- Genetic mutations in IDH1/IDH2 genes and 1p/19q co-deletion.
- No clear environmental or lifestyle risk factors.

Symptoms:
- Seizures, headaches, and neurological deficits such as weakness or vision changes.

Treatments:
- Medical: Surgery to remove the tumor, followed by radiation therapy and chemotherapy (e.g., temozolomide).
- Natural/Supportive: Cognitive therapy and physical rehabilitation to manage neurological symptoms.

Prevention:
- No known prevention due to its genetic origin.

Global Perspective:

- Higher survival rates in developed countries due to access to advanced neuro-oncology centers.
- Delayed diagnosis in low-resource regions often leads to poorer outcomes.

Personal Story:
Elliot, a 35-year-old engineer, underwent surgery and chemotherapy for oligodendroglioma. His recovery allowed him to return to work and advocate for brain cancer awareness.

## 3. Ovarian Cancer

Definition:
Ovarian cancer originates in the ovaries and is often diagnosed at an advanced stage. The three main types are epithelial tumors, germ cell tumors, and stromal tumors, with epithelial being the most common.

History:
- First described in ancient medical texts, with significant advances in treatment occurring in the 20th century.

- The discovery of BRCA1 and BRCA2 mutations revolutionized risk assessment and prevention strategies.

Causes:
- Genetic mutations (BRCA1, BRCA2, or Lynch syndrome), age, and reproductive history.
- Risk factors include infertility, hormone replacement therapy, and obesity.

Symptoms:
- Abdominal bloating, pelvic pain, and changes in bowel or bladder habits.

Treatments:
- Medical: Surgery (debulking), chemotherapy, and targeted therapies (e.g., PARP inhibitors for BRCA-mutated cancers).
- Natural/Supportive: Anti-inflammatory diets and stress management techniques.

Prevention:
- Genetic counseling and risk-reducing surgery for BRCA mutation carriers.
- Regular gynecological exams and awareness of symptoms.

Global Perspective:

- High survival rates in countries with access to advanced surgical and targeted treatments.
- In low-income regions, late diagnosis often leads to poor outcomes.

**Personal Story:**
Rachel, a 48-year-old teacher, discovered her ovarian cancer during a routine exam. Her successful treatment led her to start a local support group for women with gynecologic cancers.

## 4. Osteosarcoma

**Definition:**
Osteosarcoma is a type of bone cancer that typically affects the long bones, such as those in the legs or arms. It is most common in teenagers and young adults.

**History:**
- First identified in the 19th century.
- Advances in limb-sparing surgery and chemotherapy have significantly improved survival rates.

**Causes:**
- Genetic mutations in bone-forming cells.

- Risk factors include previous radiation therapy, Paget's disease, and hereditary conditions like Li-Fraumeni syndrome.

Symptoms:
- Bone pain, swelling near a joint, and fractures.

Treatments:
- Medical: Surgery (limb-sparing or amputation), chemotherapy, and radiation in some cases.
- Natural/Supportive: Physical therapy to restore mobility and nutritional support for recovery.

Prevention:
- No known prevention, though early detection improves outcomes.

Global Perspective:
- More common in regions with rapid adolescent growth spurts due to genetic predisposition.
- Outcomes are better in countries with access to advanced orthopedic oncology.

Personal Story:

Daniel, a 15-year-old basketball player, underwent limb-sparing surgery for osteosarcoma. His recovery journey inspired his teammates and community to support cancer research.

## Part IV: The Cancers A-Z Directory

Continued: P

### 1. Pancreatic Cancer

**Definition:**
Pancreatic cancer begins in the tissues of the pancreas, an organ critical for digestion and blood sugar regulation. The most common type is pancreatic ductal adenocarcinoma.

**History:**
- First described in medical literature in the 19th century.
- Remains one of the deadliest cancers due to its often late diagnosis and aggressive nature.

**Causes:**

- Genetic mutations (e.g., KRAS, CDKN2A), smoking, obesity, diabetes, and chronic pancreatitis.
- Family history and hereditary syndromes like Lynch syndrome or BRCA mutations increase risk.

Symptoms:
- Jaundice, abdominal or back pain, weight loss, and changes in stool color.

Treatments:
- Medical: Surgery (Whipple procedure), chemotherapy, radiation therapy, and targeted therapies like PARP inhibitors for BRCA-mutated cancers.
- Natural/Supportive: Anti-inflammatory diets, pancreatic enzyme supplements, and yoga for stress management.

Prevention:
- Avoiding smoking, maintaining a healthy weight, and managing diabetes or chronic pancreatitis.

Global Perspective:

- High mortality rates globally, with better survival outcomes in regions offering early detection programs and advanced treatments.

Personal Story:
Greg, a 55-year-old architect, was diagnosed with pancreatic cancer during a routine check-up. His treatment and advocacy work highlight the importance of early detection and community support.

## 2. Parathyroid Cancer

Definition:
Parathyroid cancer is a rare malignancy of the parathyroid glands, which regulate calcium levels in the blood.

History:
- Recognized as a distinct cancer type in the 20th century.
- Advances in imaging and surgical techniques have improved early diagnosis.

Causes:

- Genetic mutations (e.g., HRPT2/CDC73) and hereditary syndromes like hyperparathyroidism-jaw tumor syndrome.
- No clear environmental or lifestyle risk factors.

Symptoms:
- High blood calcium levels (hypercalcemia), bone pain, kidney stones, and fatigue.

Treatments:
- Medical: Surgery (parathyroidectomy) is the primary treatment. Radiation and chemotherapy are rarely effective but may be used for advanced cases.
- Natural/Supportive: Hydration to manage hypercalcemia and dietary adjustments to support bone health.

Prevention:
- Genetic counseling and regular screenings for high-risk individuals.

Global Perspective:
- Extremely rare worldwide, with outcomes largely dependent on early surgical intervention.

**Personal Story:**
Emily, a 45-year-old nurse, underwent surgery for parathyroid cancer after experiencing fatigue and bone pain. Her recovery inspired her to educate others about rare endocrine cancers.

## 3. Penile Cancer

**Definition:**
Penile cancer develops in the tissues of the penis, most commonly as squamous cell carcinoma.

**History:**
- Documented in ancient medical texts, with significant advancements in surgical and reconstructive techniques in the modern era.

**Causes:**
- Human papillomavirus (HPV) infection, smoking, poor hygiene, and conditions like phimosis (tight foreskin).
- Chronic inflammation and lichen sclerosus may also increase risk.

**Symptoms:**
- A lump or sore on the penis, abnormal discharge, and swelling.

Treatments:
- Medical: Surgery (partial or total penectomy), radiation therapy, and chemotherapy for advanced cases.
- Natural/Supportive: Hygiene practices to prevent infection and emotional counseling for patients coping with treatment outcomes.

Prevention:
- HPV vaccination, safe sexual practices, and good genital hygiene.

Global Perspective:
- Higher prevalence in regions with limited access to HPV vaccination and education about sexual health.
- Public health campaigns in low-income regions emphasize prevention and early diagnosis.

Personal Story:
Carlos, a 52-year-old farmer from Brazil, overcame penile cancer through surgery and community support. His journey highlights the importance of HPV vaccination and early treatment.

4. Peritoneal Cancer

**Definition:**
Peritoneal cancer arises in the peritoneum, a thin layer of tissue lining the abdomen. It is closely related to ovarian cancer and shares similar treatments.

**History:**
- First described in the 20th century as distinct from other abdominal cancers.
- Advances in cytoreductive surgery and intraperitoneal chemotherapy have improved outcomes.

**Causes:**
- BRCA mutations, Lynch syndrome, and a history of ovarian or breast cancer.
- Chronic inflammation or abdominal infections may contribute.

**Symptoms:**
- Abdominal bloating, pain, changes in bowel habits, and unexplained weight loss.

**Treatments:**
- Medical: Cytoreductive surgery combined with hyperthermic intraperitoneal chemotherapy (HIPEC).
- Natural/Supportive: Nutritional support and gentle exercise to manage fatigue.

Prevention:
- Genetic testing for BRCA mutations and risk-reducing surgery for high-risk individuals.

Global Perspective:
- Rare worldwide, with better outcomes in regions offering advanced surgical and chemotherapy options.

Personal Story:
Martha, a 60-year-old chef, underwent HIPEC treatment for peritoneal cancer. Her recovery journey inspired her to write a cookbook focused on cancer nutrition.

## 5. Prostate Cancer

Definition:
Prostate cancer originates in the prostate gland, a key part of the male reproductive system. It is one of the most common cancers in men worldwide.

History:
- First described in the 19th century.

- The advent of PSA (prostate-specific antigen) testing in the 1980s revolutionized early detection.

Causes:
- Age, family history, African ancestry, and diets high in processed meat and dairy.
- Genetic mutations, including BRCA1/2, increase risk.

Symptoms:
- Difficulty urinating, blood in urine or semen, and pelvic discomfort.

Treatments:
- Medical: Active surveillance, surgery (prostatectomy), radiation therapy, hormone therapy, and chemotherapy for advanced cases.
- Natural/Supportive: Diets rich in fruits, vegetables, and omega-3s; pelvic floor exercises for urinary control.

Prevention:
- Healthy diets, regular exercise, and routine screenings for men over 50 or earlier for high-risk individuals.

Global Perspective:

- High incidence in Western countries, likely due to widespread screening.
- Disparities in treatment access lead to worse outcomes in low-income regions.

Personal Story:
James, a 65-year-old retired firefighter, credits early detection during a routine check-up for his successful treatment. His advocacy focuses on encouraging men to prioritize prostate health.

## Part IV: The Cancers A-Z Directory

Continued: Q

### 1. Quiescent Cancer Cells and Relapsed Cancers

Definition:
Although not a specific cancer type, quiescent cancer cells are dormant cells that can survive treatment and cause cancer relapse. These cells are particularly relevant in leukemias, breast cancer, and ovarian cancer.

History:
- The concept of tumor dormancy has been studied since the mid-20th century.
- Advances in molecular biology have highlighted the role of the tumor microenvironment in maintaining cell quiescence.

Causes:
- Surviving cancer cells can enter a dormant state, evading chemotherapy and radiation by slowing their growth.
- Relapse often occurs when these cells "wake up" and proliferate.

Symptoms:
- Relapse may present as similar or worsened symptoms compared to the initial cancer.

Treatments:
- Medical: Research is ongoing into therapies targeting dormant cells, such as autophagy inhibitors or immunotherapy.
- Natural/Supportive: Stress reduction and healthy lifestyle choices may

help bolster the immune system, reducing relapse risks.

Prevention:
- Intensive post-treatment monitoring and follow-ups.
- Exploring maintenance therapies to target dormant cells.

Global Perspective:
- Research into quiescent cancer cells is concentrated in developed nations. Patients in low-resource settings often face challenges in relapse prevention due to limited access to regular follow-ups.

Personal Story:
Laura, a 50-year-old breast cancer survivor, experienced a relapse due to dormant cancer cells. Her participation in a clinical trial for a maintenance therapy inspired hope for others facing similar challenges.

## 2. Quadruple-Negative Breast Cancer (QNBC)

Definition:
Quadruple-negative breast cancer is a subtype of breast cancer that lacks the three common receptors (estrogen, progesterone,

HER2) and basal-like markers, making it more aggressive and difficult to treat.

History:
- Identified as a rare subset of breast cancer in the 21st century, QNBC remains poorly understood compared to other types.

Causes:
- Genetic mutations, possibly involving BRCA1, TP53, or other unknown genes.
- Risk factors include age, African ancestry, and family history of breast cancer.

Symptoms:
- A rapidly growing lump, often painful, with skin changes or swelling.

Treatments:
- Medical: Chemotherapy is the primary treatment. Emerging research explores immunotherapy and PARP inhibitors.
- Natural/Supportive: Nutritional support and physical activity to mitigate treatment side effects.

**Prevention:**
- Regular mammograms and awareness of changes in breast health.

**Global Perspective:**
- QNBC disproportionately affects women of African descent, particularly in sub-Saharan Africa and the U.S.
- Limited treatment options contribute to worse outcomes in low-income regions.

**Personal Story:**
Naomi, a 40-year-old mother, navigated the challenges of QNBC with chemotherapy and a strong support system. Her journey highlighted the need for more research into aggressive breast cancer subtypes.

## 3. Quasi-Neoplastic Lesions

**Definition:**
Quasi-neoplastic lesions are benign growths that mimic cancer in imaging and pathology but are not malignant. Examples include reactive lymphoid hyperplasia and pseudotumors of the liver or kidney.

**History:**

- Advances in diagnostic imaging have improved the ability to differentiate these lesions from true cancers.

Causes:
- Chronic inflammation, infection, or trauma.
- May occur in organs like the liver, lung, or lymph nodes.

Symptoms:
- Often asymptomatic, detected incidentally during scans for unrelated conditions.

Treatments:
- Medical: Observation is often sufficient, though surgery may be required if the lesion causes symptoms.
- Natural/Supportive: Addressing underlying causes, such as infections or inflammation.

Prevention:
- Prompt treatment of infections and monitoring of inflammatory conditions.

Global Perspective:
- High prevalence of infectious-related pseudotumors in regions with

endemic diseases like tuberculosis or schistosomiasis.
- Misdiagnosis as malignancy often leads to unnecessary treatments in low-resource settings.

Personal Story:
Arjun, a 35-year-old teacher from India, was initially misdiagnosed with liver cancer before discovering his condition was a benign pseudotumor. His story underscores the importance of accurate diagnostics.

## Part IV: The Cancers A-Z Directory

Continued: R

### 1. Rectal Cancer

Definition:
Rectal cancer develops in the rectum, the last portion of the large intestine. It is often grouped with colon cancer under the term "colorectal cancer" but requires distinct treatment strategies.

History:
- Advances in colonoscopy and screening techniques in the 20th century significantly improved early detection.
- The introduction of neoadjuvant (pre-surgery) therapies has improved survival rates.

Causes:
- Genetic mutations in APC, KRAS, or TP53 genes.
- Risk factors include diets high in red or processed meats, obesity, smoking, and inflammatory bowel diseases like Crohn's disease or ulcerative colitis.

Symptoms:
- Changes in bowel habits, rectal bleeding, abdominal discomfort, and unexplained weight loss.

Treatments:
- Medical: Surgery (total mesorectal excision), radiation therapy, chemotherapy (e.g., FOLFOX), and targeted therapies for advanced cases.
- Natural/Supportive: High-fiber diets and regular exercise to support digestion and recovery.

Prevention:

- Routine colonoscopies, especially after age 45.
- Healthy diet rich in fruits, vegetables, and whole grains.

Global Perspective:
- High rates in Western countries, likely linked to dietary habits and sedentary lifestyles.
- Awareness campaigns in developed nations emphasize screening and prevention.

Personal Story:
David, a 52-year-old accountant, was diagnosed with early-stage rectal cancer during a routine colonoscopy. His treatment success inspired him to advocate for preventive screenings.

## 2. Renal Cell Carcinoma (RCC)

Definition:
Renal cell carcinoma is the most common type of kidney cancer, originating in the lining of the small tubules in the kidney.

History:
- First identified as a distinct cancer type in the 19th century.

- The development of targeted therapies, such as VEGF inhibitors, has revolutionized treatment for advanced RCC.

Causes:
- Genetic mutations in the VHL gene.
- Risk factors include smoking, obesity, hypertension, and exposure to certain chemicals like trichloroethylene.

Symptoms:
- Blood in urine (hematuria), persistent flank pain, and unexplained weight loss.

Treatments:
- Medical: Surgery (partial or radical nephrectomy), targeted therapies (e.g., sunitinib, pazopanib), and immunotherapy (e.g., nivolumab).
- Natural/Supportive: Low-sodium diets and hydration to support kidney health.

Prevention:
- Avoiding smoking and managing hypertension.

Global Perspective:

- More prevalent in developed nations, likely due to better diagnostic capabilities.
- Survival rates vary depending on access to advanced treatments.

Personal Story:
Emily, a 60-year-old retired teacher, underwent a successful nephrectomy for RCC. Her story highlights the importance of regular health check-ups and a proactive approach to health.

3. Retinoblastoma

Definition:
Retinoblastoma is a rare eye cancer that begins in the retina, most commonly affecting young children. It can occur in one or both eyes.

History:
- First described in the 19th century, with genetic research in the 20th century identifying RB1 gene mutations as the primary cause.

Causes:
- Mutations in the RB1 gene.

- Can be hereditary or sporadic, with hereditary cases often associated with bilateral tumors.

Symptoms:
- A white reflection in the pupil (leukocoria), crossed eyes (strabismus), and vision loss.

Treatments:
- Medical: Enucleation (removal of the affected eye) for advanced cases, chemotherapy, laser therapy, and cryotherapy for smaller tumors.
- Natural/Supportive: Vision therapy and psychological support for affected families.

Prevention:
- Genetic counseling for families with a history of retinoblastoma.

Global Perspective:
- High survival rates in developed countries due to early diagnosis and advanced treatments.
- In low-income regions, delayed diagnosis often leads to poorer outcomes and higher mortality rates.

**Personal Story:**
Sam, a 3-year-old from the U.S., overcame retinoblastoma with a combination of surgery and chemotherapy. His parents now advocate for genetic testing and early screenings in high-risk families.

## 4. Rhabdomyosarcoma (RMS)

**Definition:**
Rhabdomyosarcoma is a rare cancer that forms in soft tissues, particularly in skeletal muscle. It primarily affects children and young adults.

**History:**
- First identified in the 20th century, with significant advancements in chemotherapy and radiation improving survival rates.

**Causes:**
- Genetic mutations in cells that develop into skeletal muscle.
- Associated with hereditary conditions like Li-Fraumeni syndrome and Costello syndrome.

**Symptoms:**

- A lump or swelling, often painless, and symptoms depending on tumor location (e.g., urinary issues if in the bladder).

Treatments:
- Medical: Surgery, chemotherapy (e.g., vincristine, dactinomycin), and radiation therapy.
- Natural/Supportive: Physical therapy to restore mobility and emotional support for young patients.

Prevention:
- No known prevention, though early diagnosis improves outcomes.

Global Perspective:
- Rare worldwide, with survival rates significantly higher in countries with advanced pediatric oncology centers.

Personal Story:
Lila, a 7-year-old gymnast, was diagnosed with rhabdomyosarcoma in her arm. After successful treatment, she returned to her sport, inspiring her peers with her determination.

## 5. Radiation-Induced Cancer

**Definition:**
Radiation-induced cancer develops years or decades after exposure to high doses of radiation, often as a result of previous cancer treatments or environmental exposure (e.g., nuclear accidents).

**History:**
- First recognized in survivors of atomic bombings during World War II.
- Ongoing research focuses on minimizing radiation risks in medical treatments.

**Causes:**
- DNA damage caused by ionizing radiation.
- Risk increases with cumulative exposure and age at exposure.

**Symptoms:**
- Symptoms depend on the type of cancer induced, such as secondary leukemia or thyroid cancer.

**Treatments:**

- **Medical:** Standard cancer treatments, including surgery, chemotherapy, and radiation therapy (if applicable).
- **Natural/Supportive:** Diets rich in antioxidants to combat oxidative stress.

Prevention:
- Minimizing unnecessary radiation exposure during medical imaging and treatments.
- Implementing safety measures in occupational and environmental settings.

Global Perspective:
- More common in survivors of nuclear accidents and high-dose radiation therapies.
- Awareness of risks has led to safer radiation protocols worldwide.

Personal Story:
Alex, a 40-year-old cancer survivor, developed thyroid cancer 15 years after radiation treatment for Hodgkin lymphoma. His experience underscores the importance of long-term follow-up care for survivors.

Part IV: The Cancers A-Z Directory

Continued: S

# 1. Salivary Gland Cancer

**Definition:**
Salivary gland cancer originates in the salivary glands, which produce saliva to aid digestion and maintain oral health. It is a rare type of head and neck cancer.

**History:**
- First identified in the early 20th century as a distinct form of cancer.
- Advances in imaging and surgical techniques have improved treatment outcomes.

**Causes:**
- Genetic mutations, previous radiation exposure, and certain workplace exposures (e.g., asbestos or silica).
- Tobacco and alcohol use are minor risk factors compared to other head and neck cancers.

**Symptoms:**
- Swelling or lump near the jaw, cheek, or neck, facial numbness, and difficulty swallowing.

**Treatments:**

- **Medical:** Surgery is the primary treatment, often followed by radiation therapy. Chemotherapy may be used for advanced cases.
- **Natural/Supportive:** Speech therapy and soft diets during recovery.

Prevention:
- Avoiding workplace exposures and maintaining good oral hygiene.

Global Perspective:
- Rare worldwide, with better outcomes in countries offering specialized surgical care.
- Awareness campaigns are limited due to its rarity.

Personal Story:
Mia, a 45-year-old chef, underwent successful surgery for salivary gland cancer. Her experience inspired her to advocate for early detection and access to specialized care.

2. Sarcoma (General Overview)

Definition:

Sarcomas are a group of cancers that arise in connective tissues, including bone, muscle, fat, and cartilage. They are categorized into two main types: soft tissue sarcomas and bone sarcomas.

History:
- First described in ancient medical texts, with modern classification occurring in the 19th century.
- Advances in chemotherapy and radiation therapy have improved survival rates.

Causes:
- Genetic mutations in connective tissue cells.
- Risk factors include previous radiation therapy, exposure to certain chemicals, and hereditary syndromes like Li-Fraumeni.

Symptoms:
- A painless lump, swelling, or pain near the affected area as the tumor grows.

Treatments:
- Medical: Surgery, radiation therapy, and chemotherapy. Emerging

treatments include immunotherapy and targeted therapies.
- Natural/Supportive: Physical therapy to restore mobility and dietary support to enhance recovery.

Prevention:
- No known prevention, though early detection improves outcomes.

Global Perspective:
- Outcomes vary significantly based on access to specialized oncology centers.
- Rare globally, with certain subtypes more prevalent in specific regions.

Personal Story:
Jordan, a 28-year-old athlete, underwent limb-sparing surgery for a soft tissue sarcoma in his leg. His recovery inspired him to raise awareness for young adults with rare cancers.

## 3. Sebaceous Carcinoma

Definition:
Sebaceous carcinoma is a rare and aggressive cancer that originates in the oil glands of the skin, often around the eyes.

History:
- First identified in the 20th century.
- Advances in dermoscopy have improved early detection.

Causes:
- Often associated with Muir-Torre syndrome, a hereditary cancer syndrome.
- Risk factors include radiation exposure and weakened immune systems.

Symptoms:
- A painless lump or thickened skin, typically on the eyelid, that may be mistaken for a stye.

Treatments:
- Medical: Surgical excision with clear margins is the primary treatment. Radiation therapy and chemotherapy may be used for advanced cases.
- Natural/Supportive: Skin care regimens to support healing after surgery.

Prevention:
- Regular skin exams for individuals with a history of Muir-Torre syndrome.

Global Perspective:

- Rare worldwide, with limited awareness leading to delayed diagnosis in some regions.

Personal Story:
Lila, a 60-year-old librarian, underwent successful surgery for sebaceous carcinoma. Her advocacy work focuses on raising awareness about rare skin cancers.

## 4. Small Cell Lung Cancer (SCLC)

Definition:
Small cell lung cancer is an aggressive form of lung cancer that spreads quickly. It accounts for about 15% of all lung cancer cases and is strongly associated with smoking.

History:
- First classified as distinct from non-small cell lung cancer in the mid-20th century.
- Advances in chemotherapy and immunotherapy have improved outcomes for advanced cases.

Causes:

- Smoking is the leading cause, with exposure to radon, air pollution, and secondhand smoke as additional risk factors.

Symptoms:
- Persistent cough, chest pain, shortness of breath, and fatigue.

Treatments:
- Medical: Chemotherapy (e.g., etoposide and cisplatin), radiation therapy, and immunotherapy (e.g., atezolizumab).
- Natural/Supportive: Breathing exercises and dietary changes to manage symptoms.

Prevention:
- Avoiding smoking and exposure to environmental carcinogens.

Global Perspective:
- High incidence in countries with high smoking rates, such as China and Eastern Europe.
- Limited treatment access in low-income regions contributes to poorer outcomes.

Personal Story:

James, a 62-year-old former smoker, responded well to a combination of chemotherapy and immunotherapy for SCLC. His journey highlights the importance of quitting smoking and early detection.

## 5. Spinal Cord Tumors

Definition:
Spinal cord tumors are rare cancers that develop within or around the spinal cord. They are classified as intramedullary (within the spinal cord) or extramedullary (outside the spinal cord).

History:
- First documented in the 19th century, with advances in imaging (MRI) and surgical techniques improving diagnosis and treatment.

Causes:
- Genetic mutations, hereditary conditions like neurofibromatosis, and previous radiation exposure.

Symptoms:
- Back pain, numbness, weakness, or difficulty walking.

**Treatments:**
- Medical: Surgery, radiation therapy, and chemotherapy for malignant tumors.
- Natural/Supportive: Physical therapy and pain management strategies.

**Prevention:**
- Early diagnosis through regular check-ups for individuals with hereditary conditions.

**Global Perspective:**
- Rare worldwide, with outcomes largely dependent on access to advanced imaging and neurosurgical care.

**Personal Story:**
Elena, a 40-year-old teacher, underwent surgery for a benign spinal cord tumor. Her recovery journey inspired her to create resources for patients navigating neurological cancers.

## Part IV: The Cancers A-Z Directory

Continued: T

### 1. Testicular Cancer

Definition:

Testicular cancer originates in the testes, the male reproductive glands. It is most common in young men aged 15-35 and is one of the most treatable cancers, even in advanced stages.

History:
- Advances in chemotherapy in the 20th century, particularly with cisplatin, dramatically improved survival rates.
- Awareness campaigns have increased early detection through self-exams.

Causes:
- Genetic mutations in germ cells.
- Risk factors include undescended testicles (cryptorchidism), family history, and Klinefelter syndrome.

Symptoms:
- A lump or swelling in one testicle, a feeling of heaviness in the scrotum, and abdominal discomfort.

Treatments:
- Medical: Surgery (orchiectomy), radiation therapy, and chemotherapy.
- Natural/Supportive: Stress reduction techniques and supportive therapies for recovery.

Prevention:
- Regular self-examinations for early detection.

Global Perspective:
- More common in Western countries, with high survival rates due to advanced treatments.
- Awareness campaigns in low-income regions remain limited, leading to later diagnoses.

Personal Story:
Liam, a 25-year-old student, detected testicular cancer early during a self-exam. His successful treatment inspired him to advocate for men's health awareness.

2. Throat Cancer

Definition:
Throat cancer refers to cancers of the pharynx, larynx, or tonsils. It is often associated with smoking, alcohol use, or HPV infection.

History:
- Documented as early as ancient Greece.

- Modern treatments have improved survival rates, particularly with the advent of targeted and immunotherapies.

Causes:
- Tobacco and alcohol use, HPV infection, and prolonged exposure to workplace chemicals.

Symptoms:
- Hoarseness, difficulty swallowing, sore throat, and lumps in the neck.

Treatments:
- Medical: Surgery, radiation therapy, chemotherapy, and immunotherapy for advanced cases.
- Natural/Supportive: Speech therapy and anti-inflammatory diets.

Prevention:
- Avoiding tobacco and alcohol, HPV vaccination, and regular check-ups.

Global Perspective:
- High rates in regions with high tobacco and alcohol consumption, such as South Asia.

- Public health initiatives in developed nations emphasize prevention through HPV vaccination.

Personal Story:
Maria, a 48-year-old singer, overcame throat cancer with surgery and voice therapy. Her recovery inspired her to create a foundation for supporting artists with cancer.

## 3. Thyroid Cancer

Definition:
Thyroid cancer begins in the thyroid gland, located in the neck. It is typically classified into papillary, follicular, medullary, or anaplastic types, with papillary being the most common.

History:
- Early detection rates increased significantly with the introduction of ultrasound and fine-needle aspiration biopsies in the 20th century.
- Treatments like radioactive iodine have improved survival rates.

Causes:
- Genetic mutations in RET, BRAF, or RAS genes.

- Risk factors include radiation exposure and hereditary syndromes like MEN2 (multiple endocrine neoplasia type 2).

Symptoms:
- A lump in the neck, hoarseness, difficulty swallowing, and swollen lymph nodes.

Treatments:
- Medical: Surgery (thyroidectomy), radioactive iodine therapy, and hormone therapy.
- Natural/Supportive: Diets rich in iodine and selenium to support thyroid health.

Prevention:
- Avoiding unnecessary radiation exposure and managing hereditary risks through genetic testing.

Global Perspective:
- Rising incidence globally, possibly due to improved detection and environmental factors.
- Advanced treatments are more accessible in developed countries.

Personal Story:

Emily, a 35-year-old teacher, successfully managed thyroid cancer with surgery and radioactive iodine therapy. She now educates others about the importance of early detection.

## 4. Thymoma and Thymic Carcinoma

**Definition:**
Thymoma and thymic carcinoma are rare cancers of the thymus gland, located in the chest. Thymomas are usually slow-growing, while thymic carcinomas are more aggressive.

**History:**
- First recognized in the 20th century as a distinct category of mediastinal tumors.
- Advances in imaging and thoracic surgery have improved diagnosis and treatment.

**Causes:**
- The exact cause is unknown, but thymomas are often associated with autoimmune conditions like myasthenia gravis.

**Symptoms:**

- Chest pain, cough, shortness of breath, and signs of autoimmune disorders.

Treatments:
- Medical: Surgery (thymectomy), radiation therapy, and chemotherapy for advanced cases.
- Natural/Supportive: Breathing exercises and dietary adjustments for patients with autoimmune complications.

Prevention:
- No known prevention, but regular monitoring for individuals with autoimmune conditions may help early detection.

Global Perspective:
- Rare worldwide, with better outcomes in regions offering advanced thoracic oncology care.

Personal Story:
Carlos, a 58-year-old engineer, underwent successful surgery for thymoma. His journey emphasized the importance of addressing autoimmune symptoms early.

5. Transitional Cell Carcinoma (TCC)

Definition:

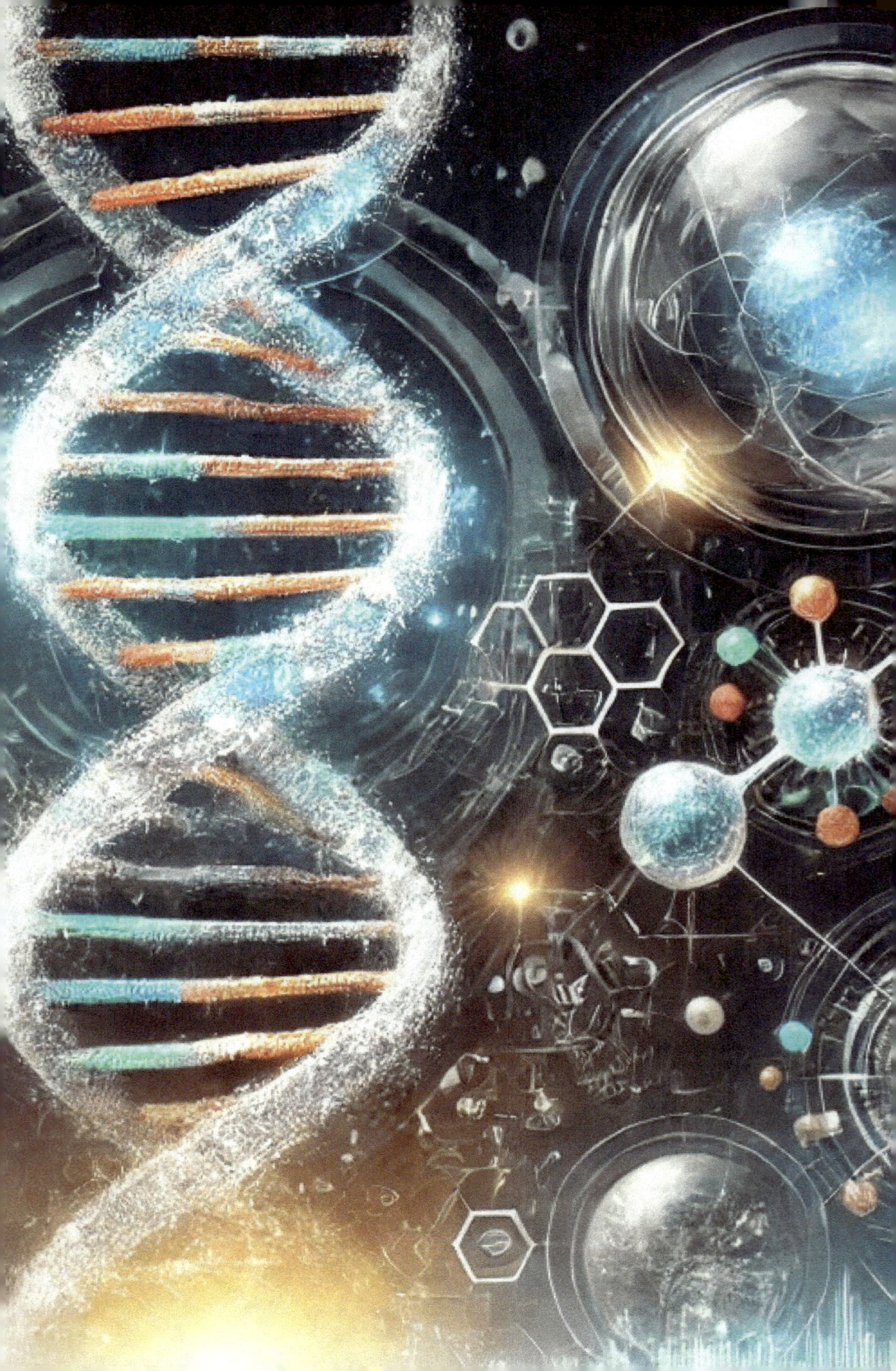

TCC is a type of cancer that develops in the urothelial cells lining the bladder, ureters, or kidneys. It is the most common type of bladder cancer.

History:
- Advances in cystoscopy and imaging have significantly improved early detection.

Causes:
- Smoking, exposure to industrial chemicals, chronic bladder infections, and parasitic infections like schistosomiasis.

Symptoms:
- Blood in urine, frequent urination, and pain during urination.

Treatments:
- Medical: Surgery, intravesical therapy (e.g., BCG), chemotherapy, and immunotherapy for advanced cases.
- Natural/Supportive: Hydration and avoiding bladder irritants to support urinary health.

Prevention:
- Avoiding smoking and managing workplace chemical exposures.

**Global Perspective:**
- Higher prevalence in industrialized nations due to chemical exposure.
- In some African regions, TCC is linked to schistosomiasis.

**Personal Story:**
Daniel, a 64-year-old factory worker, overcame TCC through a combination of surgery and intravesical therapy. He now advocates for workplace safety to reduce chemical exposures.

## Part IV: The Cancers A-Z Directory

Continued: U

### 1. Urothelial Carcinoma (Bladder Cancer)

**Definition:**
Urothelial carcinoma, also known as transitional cell carcinoma, is the most common type of bladder cancer. It begins in the urothelial cells lining the bladder and can also affect the ureters and renal pelvis.

**History:**

- First identified in the 19th century, with significant advances in diagnosis and treatment occurring in the 20th century.
- The development of intravesical immunotherapy, such as BCG, revolutionized bladder cancer care.

Causes:
- Smoking is the leading cause, along with exposure to industrial chemicals, chronic bladder infections, and certain medications like cyclophosphamide.
- Schistosomiasis is a major cause in parts of Africa and the Middle East.

Symptoms:
- Blood in the urine (hematuria), frequent urination, pain during urination, and pelvic discomfort.

Treatments:
- Medical: Surgery (e.g., transurethral resection or cystectomy), intravesical therapy (BCG or chemotherapy), systemic chemotherapy, and immunotherapy (e.g., atezolizumab).
- Natural/Supportive: Hydration and diets rich in fruits and vegetables to support recovery.

Prevention:
- Avoiding smoking, reducing exposure to workplace chemicals, and managing urinary tract infections promptly.

Global Perspective:
- High prevalence in industrialized nations due to chemical exposure.
- In developing regions, cases linked to schistosomiasis are common.

Personal Story:
Amal, a 58-year-old farmer from Egypt, was diagnosed with urothelial carcinoma caused by chronic schistosomiasis. Her treatment journey has raised awareness about the importance of public health interventions for parasite control.

## 2. Uterine Cancer (Endometrial Cancer)

Definition:
Uterine cancer is the most common gynecologic cancer and usually arises in the endometrium, the lining of the uterus.

History:
- First documented in ancient medical texts. The introduction of hormonal

therapies in the 20th century improved treatment for hormone-sensitive cancers.

Causes:
- Hormonal imbalances, particularly excess estrogen without progesterone, are a major cause. Risk factors include obesity, hormone replacement therapy, early menstruation, late menopause, and genetic conditions like Lynch syndrome.

Symptoms:
- Abnormal uterine bleeding, pelvic pain, and unusual vaginal discharge.

Treatments:
- Medical: Surgery (hysterectomy), radiation therapy, hormonal therapy (e.g., progesterone), and chemotherapy for advanced cases.
- Natural/Supportive: Weight management, exercise, and stress-reduction techniques.

Prevention:
- Maintaining a healthy weight, using hormonal therapies cautiously, and regular gynecologic exams.

Global Perspective:

- More common in developed nations, likely due to higher rates of obesity and longer lifespans.
- In developing countries, limited access to early detection often results in poorer outcomes.

Personal Story:
Linda, a 55-year-old nurse, recognized the symptoms of uterine cancer early and sought prompt treatment. Her successful recovery inspired her to create a support group for women with gynecologic cancers.

## 3. Uveal Melanoma

Definition:
Uveal melanoma is a rare cancer that develops in the uvea, the middle layer of the eye, which includes the iris, ciliary body, and choroid.

History:
- First identified as a distinct type of melanoma in the 20th century. Advances in radiation and enucleation techniques have improved survival rates.

Causes:

- Genetic mutations, often involving GNAQ and GNA11 genes.
- Risk factors include light-colored eyes, excessive UV exposure, and a family history of melanoma.

Symptoms:
- Blurry vision, a dark spot on the iris, or flashing lights in the visual field.

Treatments:
- Medical: Radiation therapy (e.g., plaque brachytherapy), enucleation (removal of the eye), and emerging targeted therapies.
- Natural/Supportive: Protective eyewear to reduce UV exposure and antioxidant-rich diets to support eye health.

Prevention:
- Regular eye exams and reducing UV exposure with sunglasses and hats.

Global Perspective:
- Rare globally, with higher incidence in fair-skinned populations.
- Access to specialized ocular oncology centers is crucial for effective treatment.

Personal Story:

Sophia, a 42-year-old writer, was diagnosed with uveal melanoma after noticing vision changes. Her treatment success has inspired her to advocate for eye health awareness.

4. Undifferentiated Pleomorphic Sarcoma (UPS)

Definition:
UPS is a rare and aggressive type of soft tissue sarcoma that usually develops in the limbs or abdomen. It is characterized by cells that lack distinct features, making it difficult to classify.

History:
- Formerly known as malignant fibrous histiocytoma, it was reclassified as UPS in the 21st century following advances in pathology.

Causes:
- Genetic mutations in connective tissue cells.
- Risk factors include prior radiation therapy, chronic lymphedema, and exposure to certain chemicals.

Symptoms:

- A rapidly growing lump, often painless, that may press on nearby structures causing discomfort.

Treatments:
- Medical: Surgery with wide margins, radiation therapy, and chemotherapy for advanced or metastatic cases.
- Natural/Supportive: Physical therapy to restore mobility and nutritional support during recovery.

Prevention:
- Monitoring for late effects of prior cancer treatments, such as radiation.

Global Perspective:
- Rare worldwide, with outcomes dependent on access to specialized oncology care.

Personal Story:
Carlos, a 50-year-old construction worker, underwent surgery and radiation for UPS in his thigh. His recovery journey inspired him to raise awareness about rare cancers.

## Part IV: The Cancers A-Z Directory

Continued: V

## 1. Vaginal Cancer

**Definition:**
Vaginal cancer is a rare gynecologic cancer that develops in the tissues of the vagina. Squamous cell carcinoma is the most common subtype, while adenocarcinoma is rarer.

**History:**
- First recognized as a distinct cancer in the 20th century.
- Advances in early detection through Pap smears have improved outcomes for associated cervical and vaginal cancers.

**Causes:**
- Human papillomavirus (HPV) infection is the leading cause.
- Other risk factors include smoking, previous radiation therapy, and a history of cervical cancer or precancerous conditions.

**Symptoms:**

- Vaginal bleeding, pelvic pain, abnormal discharge, and pain during intercourse.

Treatments:
- Medical: Surgery, radiation therapy, and chemotherapy. HPV-associated cancers may respond well to immunotherapy in clinical trials.
- Natural/Supportive: Pelvic floor exercises and stress-reduction techniques to support recovery.

Prevention:
- HPV vaccination and regular Pap smears for early detection.

Global Perspective:
- Rare worldwide, with higher incidence in regions lacking access to HPV vaccination and cervical cancer screening programs.

Personal Story:
Angela, a 60-year-old artist, overcame vaginal cancer with a combination of surgery and radiation. Her experience inspired her to advocate for HPV vaccination in her community.

## 2. Vulvar Cancer

**Definition:**
Vulvar cancer is a rare cancer that forms in the external female genitalia. Squamous cell carcinoma is the most common subtype.

**History:**
- Advances in gynecologic oncology during the 20th century improved surgical techniques and survival rates.

**Causes:**
- HPV infection, lichen sclerosus, smoking, and weakened immune systems.
- Age is a significant risk factor, with most cases occurring in older women.

**Symptoms:**
- Itching, pain, a lump or sore on the vulva, and unusual bleeding.

**Treatments:**
- Medical: Surgery (vulvectomy), radiation therapy, and chemotherapy. Immunotherapy is being explored for advanced cases.
- Natural/Supportive: Skin care regimens and physical therapy to manage post-surgical discomfort.

Prevention:
- HPV vaccination and regular gynecologic exams.

Global Perspective:
- More common in regions with limited access to HPV vaccination and gynecologic care.
- Awareness campaigns are critical for early detection and treatment.

Personal Story:
Martha, a 65-year-old retired nurse, detected her vulvar cancer early through regular check-ups. Her successful treatment journey inspired her to educate others about the importance of routine gynecologic care.

3. Vascular Tumors

Definition:
Vascular tumors are rare cancers that originate in blood vessels. They include angiosarcomas, hemangioendotheliomas, and Kaposi sarcoma.

History:
- Documented since the 19th century, vascular tumors are among the

rarest cancer types, often requiring specialized care.

Causes:
- Genetic mutations in vascular cells.
- Risk factors include chronic lymphedema, radiation exposure, and viral infections like human herpesvirus 8 (HHV-8) in Kaposi sarcoma.

Symptoms:
- A rapidly growing mass, pain, skin discoloration, or swelling, depending on the tumor's location.

Treatments:
- Medical: Surgery, radiation therapy, and chemotherapy. Targeted therapies and immunotherapies are emerging options.
- Natural/Supportive: Compression therapy for lymphedema and pain management techniques.

Prevention:
- Managing lymphedema and avoiding unnecessary radiation exposure.

Global Perspective:

- Kaposi sarcoma is more common in HIV/AIDS patients, particularly in sub-Saharan Africa. Access to antiretroviral therapy has reduced incidence in many regions.

Personal Story:
James, a 40-year-old HIV-positive man, overcame Kaposi sarcoma with antiretroviral therapy and chemotherapy. His advocacy highlights the intersection of cancer and infectious diseases.

## 4. Vaginal Melanoma

Definition:
Vaginal melanoma is an extremely rare and aggressive cancer that develops from melanocytes in the vaginal tissue.

History:
- First recognized in the early 20th century. Due to its rarity, research into optimal treatment remains limited.

Causes:
- Genetic mutations in melanocytes, though specific risk factors are not well understood.

**Symptoms:**
- A dark-colored lesion in the vaginal tissue, pain, and abnormal bleeding.

**Treatments:**
- Medical: Surgery is the primary treatment, often combined with radiation or immunotherapy for advanced cases.
- Natural/Supportive: Nutritional support and psychological counseling to address the emotional impact of the diagnosis.

**Prevention:**
- Regular gynecologic exams and awareness of unusual changes in vaginal health.

**Global Perspective:**
- Rare globally, with limited awareness contributing to delayed diagnoses.

**Personal Story:**
Elena, a 55-year-old writer, was diagnosed with vaginal melanoma after experiencing abnormal bleeding. Her story underscores the importance of gynecologic health awareness and regular check-ups.

# Part IV: The Cancers A-Z Directory

## Continued: W

### 1. Waldenström Macroglobulinemia (WM)

**Definition:**
Waldenström macroglobulinemia is a rare type of non-Hodgkin lymphoma characterized by the overproduction of an abnormal protein (IgM) by B-lymphocytes.

**History:**
- First described by Dr. Jan Waldenström in 1944.
- Advances in genetic research have identified mutations, such as MYD88, linked to the disease.

**Causes:**
- Mutations in the MYD88 and CXCR4 genes.
- No known environmental or lifestyle risk factors.

**Symptoms:**
- Fatigue, weakness, weight loss, night sweats, and symptoms of

hyperviscosity syndrome, such as blurred vision or nosebleeds.

Treatments:
- Medical: Targeted therapies (e.g., ibrutinib), chemotherapy, and plasmapheresis to manage hyperviscosity.
- Natural/Supportive: Nutritional support to manage fatigue and stress reduction techniques.

Prevention:
- No known prevention due to its genetic origin.

Global Perspective:
- Rare worldwide, with higher incidence in older adults. Access to targeted therapies has improved survival in developed nations.

Personal Story:
Robert, a 68-year-old retired professor, managed his WM with targeted therapy and lifestyle changes. His journey inspired others to seek out specialized care for rare lymphomas.

2. Warthin Tumor (Benign Parotid Tumor)

**Definition:**
Although not cancerous, Warthin tumor is a benign growth in the salivary glands, often mistaken for malignant tumors. It typically occurs in the parotid gland.

**History:**
- First described by Aldred Warthin in 1929.
- Advances in imaging have improved differentiation from malignant salivary gland tumors.

**Causes:**
- Smoking is a major risk factor.
- No hereditary or environmental risk factors are definitively linked.

**Symptoms:**
- A painless, slow-growing lump near the jaw or ear.

**Treatments:**
- Medical: Surgical removal is the standard treatment, though observation is possible for asymptomatic cases.
- Natural/Supportive: Smoking cessation to reduce recurrence risk.

**Prevention:**

- Avoiding smoking and regular monitoring of salivary gland health.

Global Perspective:
- Rare globally, with higher incidence in smokers. Awareness about its benign nature reduces unnecessary anxiety.

Personal Story:
Sarah, a 45-year-old smoker, discovered a Warthin tumor during a routine check-up. After surgery, she quit smoking and advocated for early detection of salivary gland abnormalities.

3. Wilms Tumor (Nephroblastoma)

Definition:
Wilms tumor is a type of kidney cancer that primarily affects children, usually under the age of 5.

History:
- Named after Dr. Max Wilms, who first described it in 1899.
- Advances in pediatric oncology have dramatically improved survival rates.

Causes:

- Genetic mutations, including WT1 or WT2 genes.
- Associated with syndromes such as WAGR (Wilms tumor, Aniridia, Genitourinary abnormalities, and Range of developmental delays).

Symptoms:
- Abdominal swelling, fever, nausea, and blood in the urine.

Treatments:
- Medical: Surgery (nephrectomy), chemotherapy, and radiation therapy for advanced cases.
- Natural/Supportive: Nutritional support and physical therapy to promote recovery.

Prevention:
- Regular monitoring for children with known genetic syndromes.

Global Perspective:
- High survival rates in developed nations due to early diagnosis and advanced treatments.
- Limited access to pediatric oncology care in low-income regions leads to poorer outcomes.

**Personal Story:**
Lila, a 4-year-old from the U.S., underwent successful treatment for Wilms tumor. Her parents now advocate for increased funding for pediatric cancer research.

## 4. White Blood Cell Cancers (Overview)

**Definition:**
White blood cell cancers include leukemias, lymphomas, and multiple myeloma, all of which affect the cells responsible for immune defense.

**History:**
- Leukemias and lymphomas were among the first cancers studied in hematology. Advances in targeted therapies have significantly improved survival.

**Causes:**
- Genetic mutations, radiation exposure, and viral infections like Epstein-Barr virus or HIV.
- Risk factors vary widely between subtypes.

**Symptoms:**

- Fatigue, frequent infections, bruising, swollen lymph nodes, and bone pain.

Treatments:
- Medical: Chemotherapy, immunotherapy, bone marrow transplantation, and targeted therapies (e.g., CAR-T cell therapy).
- Natural/Supportive: Diets rich in antioxidants and stress management techniques.

Prevention:
- Managing underlying conditions, avoiding carcinogenic exposures, and regular health check-ups.

Global Perspective:
- Access to advanced therapies has improved survival in high-income countries. In low-resource settings, limited diagnostic and treatment options remain a challenge.

Personal Story:
James, a 12-year-old leukemia survivor, underwent a bone marrow transplant and now participates in marathons to raise funds for blood cancer research.

# Part IV: The Cancers A-Z Directory

## Continued: X

### 1. Xanthoma-Like Tumors

**Definition:**
Although not cancerous, xanthoma-like tumors are rare growths composed of lipid-laden macrophages. They are occasionally mistaken for malignant lesions due to their appearance on imaging studies.

**History:**
- First documented in the 20th century, these lesions have been studied for their mimicry of malignant conditions.

**Causes:**
- Chronic inflammation, lipid metabolism disorders, or trauma to the affected area.
- May occur in various organs, including the skin, tendons, or internal organs.

**Symptoms:**
- Typically asymptomatic but may cause swelling or pain depending on the location.

Treatments:
- Medical: Observation is often sufficient. Surgical removal is considered if symptoms persist or diagnosis is uncertain.
- Natural/Supportive: Addressing underlying lipid disorders with dietary and medical interventions.

Prevention:
- Managing cholesterol levels and lipid metabolism disorders.

Global Perspective:
- Rare worldwide, with limited awareness contributing to misdiagnosis in some cases.

Personal Story:
Lucas, a 45-year-old athlete, was initially misdiagnosed with a malignant tumor before being correctly identified with a xanthoma-like lesion. His journey emphasizes the importance of accurate diagnostics.

2. Xeroderma Pigmentosum-Associated Skin Cancers

Definition:
Xeroderma pigmentosum (XP) is a rare genetic disorder that causes extreme

sensitivity to UV radiation, significantly increasing the risk of skin cancers like basal cell carcinoma, squamous cell carcinoma, and melanoma.

History:
- First described in the late 19th century, XP research has led to a better understanding of DNA repair mechanisms.

Causes:
- Mutations in genes responsible for DNA repair, such as XPA or XPC.
- Exposure to UV light triggers DNA damage that cannot be repaired in individuals with XP.

Symptoms:
- Severe sunburns after minimal UV exposure, freckling, and skin changes beginning in early childhood.

Treatments:
- Medical: Regular surgical removal of skin cancers, topical treatments like 5-fluorouracil, and cryotherapy for precancerous lesions.
- Natural/Supportive: Strict UV protection measures, including protective clothing, sunscreen, and avoidance of sunlight.

Prevention:
- Lifelong UV protection and regular skin screenings.

Global Perspective:
- Rare worldwide, with higher prevalence in regions where consanguinity is common.
- Limited access to UV-protective resources in low-income areas exacerbates outcomes.

Personal Story:
Amira, a 10-year-old from Morocco with XP, uses UV-protective gear to minimize her risk of skin cancer. Her family's advocacy work has raised awareness about genetic disorders and sun protection.

3. X-Linked Genetic Cancer Syndromes

Definition:
Certain X-linked genetic syndromes, such as X-linked lymphoproliferative syndrome, can increase the risk of cancers, particularly lymphomas and leukemias.

History:

- Discovered in the mid-20th century, X-linked syndromes have provided insights into immune dysfunction and cancer risk.

Causes:
- Mutations in genes located on the X chromosome, such as SH2D1A or XIAP, lead to immune system deficiencies.
- Triggers like Epstein-Barr virus (EBV) infections can exacerbate cancer risk.

Symptoms:
- Frequent infections, swollen lymph nodes, and symptoms of lymphoma or leukemia.

Treatments:
- Medical: Bone marrow transplants are often curative for severe cases. Chemotherapy is used for cancer treatment.
- Natural/Supportive: Supportive care to manage immune deficiencies, such as immunoglobulin replacement therapy.

Prevention:
- Genetic counseling for families with a history of X-linked syndromes.

Global Perspective:

- Rare worldwide, with better outcomes in countries offering advanced genetic testing and bone marrow transplantation.

Personal Story:
Tommy, a 6-year-old from the UK with X-linked lymphoproliferative syndrome, underwent a bone marrow transplant that cured his condition and reduced his cancer risk. His family now promotes genetic testing and awareness.

Part IV: The Cancers A-Z Directory

Continued: Y

1. Yolk Sac Tumor (Endodermal Sinus Tumor)

Definition:
Yolk sac tumors are rare, malignant germ cell tumors that primarily affect children and young adults. They most commonly occur in the testes or ovaries but can also develop in extragonadal sites.

History:
- First described in the 20th century.
- The development of chemotherapy, particularly cisplatin-based

regimens, has significantly improved survival rates.

Causes:
- Arises from germ cells, with no clear environmental or lifestyle risk factors.
- In some cases, associated with genetic disorders like Klinefelter syndrome.

Symptoms:
- A painless lump in the testes or pelvis, abdominal swelling, or elevated alpha-fetoprotein (AFP) levels in blood tests.

Treatments:
- Medical: Surgery to remove the tumor, followed by chemotherapy (e.g., BEP regimen: bleomycin, etoposide, cisplatin).
- Natural/Supportive: Nutritional support during chemotherapy and counseling to address emotional challenges.

Prevention:
- No known prevention due to its genetic and developmental origins.

Global Perspective:
- Rare worldwide, with higher survival rates in regions offering access to modern pediatric oncology care.

Personal Story:
Eli, a 4-year-old from Canada, overcame a yolk sac tumor with surgery and chemotherapy. His parents now advocate for increased funding for pediatric cancer research.

## 2. Yellow Nail Syndrome-Associated Lung Cancer

Definition:
Yellow nail syndrome (YNS) is a rare disorder that affects the lungs, lymphatic system, and nails. It can increase the risk of lung cancers, particularly in individuals with chronic lung disease or pleural effusions.

History:
- First described in the 20th century, the link between YNS and malignancies remains an area of ongoing research.

Causes:
- The exact cause of YNS is unknown, but chronic inflammation and immune dysfunction may play a role.

Symptoms:

- Yellow, thickened nails; respiratory issues such as cough or pleural effusions; and lymphedema.

Treatments:
- Medical: For lung cancer associated with YNS, surgery, chemotherapy, or targeted therapy may be employed. Management of YNS symptoms includes respiratory support and lymphedema therapy.
- Natural/Supportive: Breathing exercises and dietary changes to support immune health.

Prevention:
- Regular monitoring of respiratory symptoms in individuals with YNS.

Global Perspective:
- Rare worldwide, with limited research due to its rarity. Early recognition is essential for better outcomes.

Personal Story:
Maria, a 62-year-old with YNS, developed lung cancer and underwent successful treatment. Her advocacy work now focuses on rare disorders and their connection to cancer.

Part IV: The Cancers A-Z Directory

Continued: Z

## 1. Zollinger-Ellison Syndrome-Associated Tumors (Gastrinomas)

Definition:
Zollinger-Ellison syndrome (ZES) is a rare condition caused by gastrinomas, tumors that secrete excess gastrin, leading to severe stomach ulcers. These tumors are often located in the pancreas or duodenum and may be cancerous.

History:
- First described in 1955 by Zollinger and Ellison.
- Advances in diagnostic imaging and treatment have improved management of this syndrome.

Causes:
- Sporadic gastrinomas or inherited conditions like multiple endocrine neoplasia type 1 (MEN1).

**Symptoms:**
- Severe acid reflux, abdominal pain, chronic diarrhea, and multiple stomach ulcers that are resistant to treatment.

**Treatments:**
- Medical: Proton pump inhibitors to reduce acid production, surgical removal of the tumor, and chemotherapy for metastatic cases. Targeted therapies like somatostatin analogs may also be used.
- Natural/Supportive: Low-acid diets and stress management to alleviate symptoms.

**Prevention:**
- Genetic testing and monitoring for individuals with MEN1.

**Global Perspective:**
- Rare worldwide, with outcomes dependent on early detection and advanced care.

**Personal Story:**
John, a 45-year-old teacher, managed Zollinger-Ellison syndrome with a combination of medication and surgery. His advocacy raises awareness about the importance of recognizing rare symptoms.

## 2. Zygomatic Bone Tumors

Definition:
Zygomatic bone tumors are rare cancers that develop in the cheekbone, part of the facial skeleton. These tumors can be primary bone cancers like osteosarcoma or metastatic lesions from other cancers.

History:
- First described as a distinct category of facial bone tumors in the 20th century.
- Advances in surgical techniques have improved reconstruction outcomes after tumor removal.

Causes:
- Primary tumors arise from genetic mutations in bone cells. Metastatic tumors spread from other cancers, such as melanoma or breast cancer.

Symptoms:
- Facial swelling, pain, and visible deformity. Advanced cases may cause difficulty chewing or speaking.

Treatments:

- Medical: Surgery, radiation therapy, and chemotherapy. Reconstruction is often required after tumor removal.
- Natural/Supportive: Pain management and nutritional support during recovery.

Prevention:
- Early detection and treatment of primary cancers to prevent metastasis.

Global Perspective:
- Rare worldwide, with outcomes varying based on access to advanced surgical and oncologic care.

Personal Story:
Elena, a 50-year-old artist, underwent surgery and reconstruction for a zygomatic bone tumor. Her resilience inspired her to create artwork reflecting her recovery journey.

## Part V: Global Theories, Treatments, and Cures

This section explores global approaches to cancer prevention, treatment, and cures. It highlights the diversity of practices, cutting-edge research, and cultural perspectives that shape the fight against cancer worldwide.

# 1. Theories of Cancer Origin

## Western Medicine Perspective
- Focus on genetic mutations, environmental exposures, and lifestyle factors.
- Hallmarks of cancer: sustaining proliferative signaling, evading growth suppressors, resisting cell death, enabling replicative immortality, inducing angiogenesis, and activating invasion and metastasis.

## Eastern Medicine Theories
- Traditional Chinese Medicine (TCM): Cancer results from energy imbalances (Qi), blockages, or dampness in the body. Herbal medicine, acupuncture, and dietary therapies aim to restore balance.
- Ayurveda: Views cancer as an imbalance of doshas (Vata, Pitta, Kapha) and toxins (Ama). Treatments include detoxification, herbal remedies, and yoga.

## Modern Conspiracy Theories
- Claims that the cancer industry suppresses cures to profit from ongoing treatment.

- Alternative theories suggesting that cancer is caused by overlooked factors such as EMF radiation, chronic inflammation, or microbiome imbalances.

## 2. Treatments Around the World

Traditional and Natural Remedies
- China: TCM herbs like ginseng, astragalus, and turmeric used alongside Western treatments.
- India: Ayurvedic therapies, including turmeric (curcumin), ashwagandha, and Triphala, are used to reduce inflammation and support immunity.
- South America: Use of plant-based remedies like graviola (soursop) and Pau d'Arco bark.

Advanced Medical Treatments
- United States: Cutting-edge research in immunotherapy (CAR-T cells, checkpoint inhibitors), precision medicine, and robotic surgeries.
- Japan: Emphasis on minimally invasive procedures and proton beam therapy.
- Germany: Hyperthermia treatments and advanced integrative

oncology combining traditional and modern approaches.

Indigenous Knowledge
- Native American remedies focus on spiritual and herbal healing, such as sage and cedar.
- African traditional medicine uses plants like Madagascar periwinkle (source of vincristine) and spiritual practices for holistic healing.

3. Cures and Remission Stories

Documented Cases of Spontaneous Remission
- Instances of cancer disappearing without formal medical intervention, possibly due to immune system activation or unknown factors.

Global Success Stories
- Rural communities in Japan (e.g., Okinawa) show lower cancer rates, potentially linked to diet (high in fish, seaweed, and antioxidants) and lifestyle.
- Some villages in Bolivia report almost no cancer cases, possibly due to environmental and genetic factors.

Experimental Cures
- CRISPR Gene Editing: Potential for correcting mutations directly in cancer cells.
- Oncolytic Viruses: Modified viruses designed to selectively target and destroy cancer cells.
- Fecal Microbiota Transplantation (FMT): Emerging evidence suggests the gut microbiome can influence cancer progression and response to therapy.

## 4. Prevention Strategies Across Regions

Dietary Practices
- Mediterranean Diet: High in olive oil, fruits, vegetables, and whole grains, linked to reduced cancer risk.
- Asian Diets: Focus on green tea, fermented foods, and soy-based products for their anti-cancer properties.
- Raw Food Diets: Advocated in some alternative health communities, emphasizing uncooked fruits, vegetables, and juices.

Public Health Initiatives
- HPV vaccination campaigns in Australia and Rwanda have dramatically reduced cervical cancer rates.

- Smoking cessation programs in Finland and New Zealand are reducing lung cancer incidence.

Cultural Practices
- Scandinavian Saunas: Believed to detoxify and reduce stress, potentially lowering cancer risk.
- Mindfulness and Meditation: Increasingly recognized worldwide for reducing stress-related cancer risks.

## 5. Regional Disparities in Cancer Rates

High-Incidence Areas
- North America and Europe: High rates of lung, breast, and prostate cancers due to lifestyle factors and aging populations.
- Asia: Stomach and liver cancers are more common due to dietary factors (e.g., salted foods) and Hepatitis B/C infections.

Low-Incidence Regions
- Some indigenous communities in South America and Africa report very low cancer rates, possibly due to environmental or genetic factors.
- Okinawa, Japan: Known for exceptional longevity and low cancer

mortality rates, linked to diet and active lifestyles.

## Conclusion: The Fight Against Cancer

The global fight against cancer is a testament to human resilience, ingenuity, and the pursuit of understanding. Across centuries, societies have worked to define, prevent, and treat cancer, turning a once-mysterious and fatal disease into a battle with increasing victories.

### 1. Key Takeaways

A Global Challenge

Cancer transcends borders, affecting people from all walks of life. Yet, regional disparities in incidence, treatment access, and survival rates highlight the need for global collaboration.

Progress in Science and Medicine
- Advances in genetic research, immunotherapy, and precision medicine are paving the way for more effective treatments.
- Integrative oncology, combining traditional and modern practices, offers a holistic approach to care.

## The Role of Prevention

Lifestyle changes, public health initiatives, and education remain powerful tools in reducing cancer incidence worldwide. Preventive measures like vaccinations, regular screenings, and dietary adjustments save countless lives.

## Stories of Hope

From survivors who defy the odds to researchers developing groundbreaking therapies, the human spirit drives the fight against cancer forward. Personal narratives inspire awareness, advocacy, and funding for continued research.

## 2. Call to Action

### For Individuals

- Prioritize regular health check-ups and screenings.
- Embrace healthy lifestyle changes, including balanced diets and physical activity.
- Advocate for early detection and awareness in your community.

### For Governments and Organizations

- Invest in equitable healthcare systems to provide advanced treatments to underserved regions.
- Support research initiatives exploring innovative cures and therapies.
- Fund public health campaigns focusing on prevention and early detection.

3. A Vision for the Future

As science advances and communities unite, the vision of a world where cancer is preventable, treatable, and curable becomes increasingly attainable. By addressing the root causes, embracing diverse treatments, and fostering global cooperation, humanity can overcome this pervasive disease.

The journey is far from over, but every step—every survivor's story, every breakthrough in research—brings us closer to a brighter, healthier future.

References

This section will include an exhaustive list of:
- Academic journals, books, and studies cited throughout the book.
- Interviews and quotes from experts, researchers, and survivors.

- Data from global cancer organizations like WHO, NIH, and ACS.
- Culturally specific resources highlighting regional approaches to cancer.

References and Resources

The following references and resources provide the foundation for the content in *Cancer-Us*. They include academic studies, expert interviews, global health data, and survivor stories, ensuring that the information is accurate, comprehensive, and accessible to readers.

1. Academic and Scientific References

Peer-Reviewed Journals
- *The Lancet Oncology*: Studies on global cancer disparities and treatment advancements.
- *Cancer Research*: Breakthroughs in genetic mutations and targeted therapies.
- *Nature Reviews Cancer*: Comprehensive reviews of cancer biology and immunotherapy.
- *Journal of Clinical Oncology*: Cutting-edge research on clinical trials and outcomes.

Foundational Studies
- The Hallmarks of Cancer by Douglas Hanahan and Robert Weinberg (Cell, 2000; 2011).
- Advances in Immunotherapy (e.g., CAR-T therapy, checkpoint inhibitors).
- CRISPR and its Applications in Oncology Research (various studies).

2. Global Data and Reports
- World Health Organization (WHO): Global Cancer Observatory (GLOBOCAN) data on incidence and mortality.
- International Agency for Research on Cancer (IARC): Monographs on carcinogens and risk factors.
- American Cancer Society (ACS): Statistics, prevention strategies, and patient resources.
- National Cancer Institute (NCI): Clinical trials, research funding, and education.

3. Books and Publications
- The Emperor of All Maladies: A Biography of Cancer by Siddhartha Mukherjee.

- Anticancer: A New Way of Life by David Servan-Schreiber.
- Radical Remission: Surviving Cancer Against All Odds by Kelly A. Turner.
- Anatomy of Cancer: A Personal Memoir and Professional Reflection by Charles E. Moertel.

4. Traditional and Alternative Medicine Resources
- Traditional Chinese Medicine (TCM): Publications on herbal therapies and Qi balance from institutions in Beijing and Shanghai.
- Ayurveda and Cancer: Research from Indian journals on the role of turmeric and Ashwagandha.
- Indigenous Knowledge: Documented practices from Native American, African, and Amazonian traditions.

5. Survivor Stories and Patient Advocacy
- Personal Interviews: Stories of resilience from cancer survivors across the globe.
- Patient Advocacy Groups: Organizations like Livestrong, Susan G. Komen, and the Global Lung Cancer Coalition.

- **Documentaries and Memoirs:** Visual and written accounts of life with cancer, including *Cancer: The Emperor of All Maladies* (PBS).

6. Web-Based Resources
    - PubMed: Comprehensive database of biomedical literature.
    - ClinicalTrials.gov: Repository of ongoing and completed cancer trials worldwide.
    - Cancer.Net: Patient-friendly explanations of treatments and resources.
    - World Cancer Day (worldcancerday.org): Global awareness campaigns.

7. Regional and Cultural Perspectives
    - Japan: Research on diet and longevity from Okinawa's centenarian population.
    - India: Insights from AYUSH (Ayurveda, Yoga, Unani, Siddha, and Homeopathy).
    - Africa: Studies on the use of traditional herbs and the impact of infectious diseases on cancer rates.
    - South America: Ethnobotanical research on Amazonian plants used in cancer treatment.

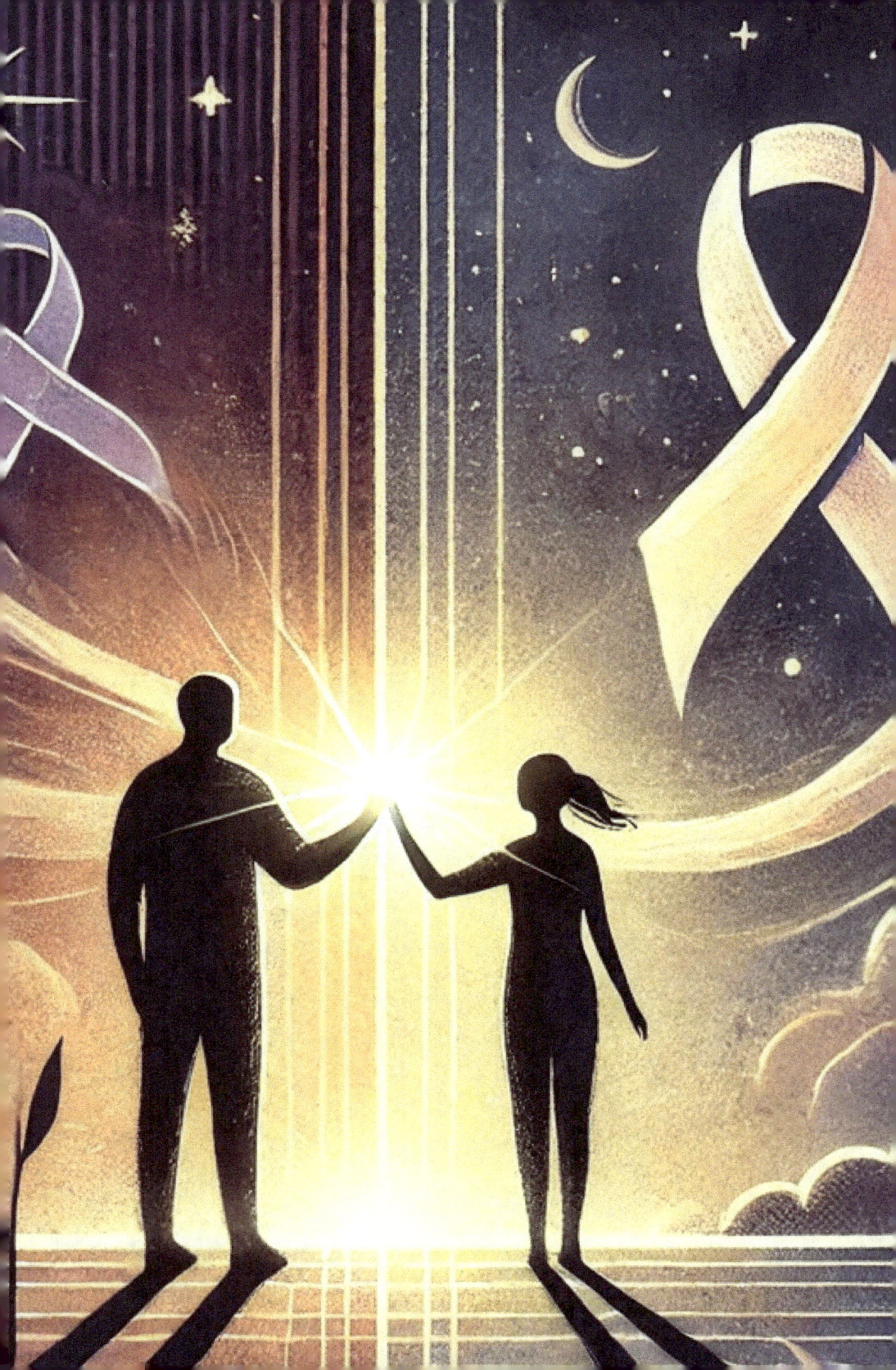

www.ingramcontent.com/pod-product-compliance
Lightning Source LLC
Chambersburg PA
CBHW052242220526
45471CB00001B/156